Anin
Veter

The Universities Federation for Animal Welfare

UFAW, founded in 1926, is an internationally recognised, independent, scientific and educational animal welfare charity that promotes high standards of welfare for farm, companion, laboratory and captive wild animals, and for those animals with which we interact in the wild. It works to improve animals' lives by:

- Funding and publishing developments in the science and technology that underpin advances in animal welfare;
- Promoting education in animal care and welfare;
- Providing information, organising meetings and publishing books, videos, articles, technical reports and the journal *Animal Welfare*;
- Providing expert advice to government departments and other bodies and helping to draft and amend laws and guidelines;
- Enlisting the energies of animal keepers, scientists, veterinarians, lawyers and others who care about animals.

'Improvements in the care of animals are not now likely to come of their own accord, merely by wishing them: there must be research ... and it is in sponsoring research of this kind, and making its results widely known, that UFAW performs one of its most valuable services.'

Sir Peter Medawar CBE FRS, 8th May 1957
Nobel Laureate (1960), Chairman of the UFAW Scientific Advisory Committee (1951–1962)

UFAW relies on the generosity of the public through legacies and donations to carry out its work, improving the welfare of animals now and in the future. For further information about UFAW and how you can help promote and support its work, please contact us at the following address:

Universities Federation for Animal Welfare
The Old School, Brewhouse Hill, Wheathampstead, Herts AL4 8AN, UK
Tel: 01582 831818 Fax: 01582 831414 Website: www.ufaw.org.uk
Email: ufaw@ufaw.org.uk

UFAW's aim regarding the UFAW/Wiley-Blackwell Animal Welfare book series is to promote interest and debate in the subject and to disseminate information relevant to improving the welfare of kept animals and of those harmed in the wild through human agency. The books in this series are the works of their authors, and the views they express do not necessarily reflect the views of UFAW.

Animal Welfare in Veterinary Practice

James Yeates

BVSc, BSc (Hons), DWEL, Dip-ECAWBM (WSEL),
PhD, MRCVS
Honorary Lecturer, University of Bristol
and Chief Veterinary Officer, RSPCA, Sussex, UK

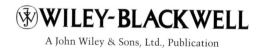
WILEY-BLACKWELL

A John Wiley & Sons, Ltd., Publication

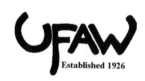
Established 1926

Registered Office
John Wiley & Sons, Ltd, The Atrium, Southern Gate, Chichester, West Sussex, PO19 8SQ, UK

Editorial Offices
9600 Garsington Road, Oxford, OX4 2DQ, UK
The Atrium, Southern Gate, Chichester, West Sussex, PO19 8SQ, UK
2121 State Avenue, Ames, Iowa 50014–8300, USA

For details of our global editorial offices, for customer services and for information about how
to apply for permission to reuse the copyright material in this book please see our website at
www.wiley.com/wiley-blackwell.

Library of Congress Cataloging-in-Publication Data

Yeates, James, 1980–
    Animal welfare in veterinary practice / James Yeates.
      p. ; cm. – (UFAW animal welfare series)
    Includes bibliographical references and index.
    ISBN 978-1-4443-3487-6 (pbk. : alk. paper)   1. Animal welfare.   2. Veterinary medicine.
I. Universities Federation for Animal Welfare.
II. Title.   III. Series: UFAW animal welfare series.
    [DNLM: 1. Animal Welfare.   2. Veterinary Medicine–ethics. HV 4708]
    HV4708.Y43 2013
    636.089–dc23
                                                        2012031336

A catalogue record for this book is available from the British Library.

Wiley also publishes its books in a variety of electronic formats. Some content that appears in print
may not be available in electronic books.

Cover image: courtesy of James Yeates
Cover design by Sandra Heath

Set in 10/12.5pt Sabon by SPi Publisher Services, Pondicherry, India
Printed in Singapore by Ho Printing Singapore Pte Ltd

1   2013

Contents

Foreword

'The veterinary profession is the ultimate arbiter and protector of animal welfare'. This is a mantra I've heard many times, usually from the mouths of veterinary surgeons. Is this an objective statement of fact or a means of professional self-protection? It's certainly a laudable aspirational goal; but do veterinary practitioners work to fulfil it, or do they merely hold on to it to displace the disappointment of everyday reality that animal keepers inevitably hold the balance of power reducing the influential scope of the individual vet and the wider profession?

The UK's Royal College of Veterinary Surgeons 2012 Code of Professional Conduct includes the following declaration made by all veterinary surgeons as a condition of admission: '*I PROMISE AND SOLEMNLY DECLARE that I will pursue the work of my profession with integrity and accept my responsibilities to the public, my clients, the profession and the Royal College of Veterinary Surgeons, and that, ABOVE ALL, my constant endeavour will be to ensure the health and welfare of animals committed to my care*'. The upper case letters are not my addition; '*ABOVE ALL*', UK veterinary surgeons must work to ensure animal health and welfare, a standard that fits well with the aspiration described above. Many other countries have oaths for their veterinary surgeons similarly stating the importance of animal welfare, so that this should be the case seems not to be in contention. The question remains – what does the profession actually do to achieve it?

That the veterinary profession lost ground in the advancement of animal welfare science over a number of years is beyond doubt. At practitioner level, concentrating on the immediacy of ill-health as the prime indicator of good or bad welfare could almost be viewed as the course of least resistance and it is easy to see how the profession fell into this trap while science moved on around it. Good or bad animal health is undoubtedly an indicator of good or bad animal welfare, but assessing animal welfare is so much more than merely benchmarking animal health. This failing has thankfully been recognised and there is much work going on to redress the balance.

To achieve real improvements in animal welfare, veterinary practitioners need appropriate tools to influence the behaviour of animal keepers. These are not simply those of recognition, diagnosis and measurement familiar to those in practice, they also include objective and productive methods of assessment, reflection and communication techniques that have been less commonly adopted. This book describes the concept of a 'welfare account' where each veterinary surgeon (and indeed the veterinary profession collectively and each client/animal keeper) should manage their account with deposits and withdrawals in a similar way to a monetary bank account, aiming to remain in credit and avoid being overdrawn with negative welfare outcomes by adapting old tools and adopting new ones. It points practitioners in a direction to deliver the RCVS oath, noting pragmatically that 'Practitioners should not be ashamed of the fact that they make money, enjoy their job, learn from their previous cases, maintain good public relations and have not been sued, when these are achieved as a **side effect** of welfare-focused veterinary work'. A welcome recognition of the place in which practitioners find themselves in what they would describe as the real world.

I first met James Yeates when he attended a British Veterinary Association: Animal Welfare Foundation course for final year undergraduate veterinary students in 2003, aimed at addressing everyday animal welfare challenges that occur in first opinion practice and achieving positive outcomes. His contributions to discussion were expansive, well thought through and stimulatory in a way I had not seen in delegates at this course before or since. In this book it is encouraging to see that this refreshing and challenging approach has been further developed.

When attempting to act as the final arbiter and guardian of animal welfare, practitioners should reflect on what they do in their every day working life that achieves that aim. This book provides tools to realise the aspiration.

Carl Padgett, BVMS, CertCHP, MRCVS

Foreword

Fresh-faced, enthusiastic but naive veterinary students often passionately believe that they can make a difference and improve welfare of animals committed to their care. Thankfully, provided we equip students with the necessary knowledge base and skills, then during their professional career they can make a positive impact on the lives of their patients and their patients' owners. This positive influence and the generally high esteem placed on the profession by the general public ensure the professional life of a veterinary surgeon is still hugely rewarding.

However, scratch beneath the surface and many veterinary surgeons are frustrated by their lack of ability to persuade owners to do the right thing for their animals. The simple truth is that owners usually retain the day to day responsibility for the care of their animals. Therefore, often the veterinary surgeon's ability to improve welfare depends more on their ability to influence client behaviour than on any clinical knowledge. Whilst waiting for Utopia, we probably ought to also recognise that not everybody is working towards the same common goals. Concern for animal welfare has to compete with other values ranging from the rational, such as the sustainability of our rural communities, to the irrational, such as the aesthetic considerations of the show ring.

This book takes a very positive and pragmatic approach to this challenge. The overriding theme is 'how can the veterinary profession promote better animal welfare'? Somebody not familiar with the veterinary profession would perhaps wonder how a whole book can be dedicated to this topic. Surely that is fundamental to what veterinary surgeons do every day? The critical proposition raised by this book is that the veterinary profession should review how it can deliver on this assumed animal advocate role. Society expects the profession to promote the interests of animals. What does that actually mean in practice?

Refreshingly James Yeates does not dwell on the academic debate over welfare definitions, rather he refers to the 'vague' concern for animals' interests. He does, however, move the debate forward on several different counts including welfare assessment, consideration of owners' interests, and the potential relationships between owners and veterinary professionals.

In Chapter 2, James states that owners are part of the problem as well as part of the solution. I have also heard it stated that the veterinary profession is also part of the problem as well as the solution. During discussions of contentious animal welfare issues, I have often felt that veterinary surgeons are all too willing to take on the devil's advocate position. It sometimes seems easier to represent the views of their most sceptical client rather than try to promote a more pro-active welfare-focused view. This book tackles these issues head on and attempts to provide solutions. It should be read widely within the profession and should stimulate further reflection and discussion upon the profession's assumed role as an animal advocate.

David Main, BVetMed, PhD, CertVR, DWEL,
DipECAWBM (AWSEL), MRCVS

Preface

Veterinary professionals are concerned about animal welfare and want to make a difference. This concern for animals is why most of us joined, stay in and enjoy the profession. There is an enormous potential to improve animals' welfare using the knowledge, enthusiasm, intelligence and compassion of the veterinary professionals. This is a global opportunity, although the statuses of animals and the veterinary professions differ between countries and areas. This potential has begun to be increasingly captured and developed, and there are many more opportunities that we can fulfil as the profession develops its role in animal welfare in all societies. Many other people are doing very many things. This book hopes to contribute to, stimulate and assist with realising these opportunities.

At the same time, concern for animals is why many people dislike practice or leave the profession. Some of the most intelligent, caring and concerned people stop helping animals, precisely because they are concerned about animals. This attrition may be due to those veterinary professionals who decide to specialise in animal welfare become animal welfare scientists. Or it may be due to the frustration borne of the seeming endlessness of welfare problems, with each day bringing more of the same problems despite the work of the day before.

Veterinary professionals need tools to deal with obstacles such as financial limitations, lack of time, clients' resistance and owners' non-compliance. So this book aims at providing practical and realistic methods for working with owners to improve patients' welfare, within the realistic constraints of everyday practice. Veterinary professionals also need to work within the law so, while nothing in this book should be taken as legal guidance, it tries to provide advice that is useful for work within many jurisdictions. The book also tries to be realistic about what busy veterinary professionals can read, by summarising other research, including only vital references, providing further reading sources and recapping key points at the end of each chapter. Where there are easy and proven answers, they are given. Where there are not easy options, the book gives new ideas and general advice to help each veterinary professional to make their personal decision about their own cases.

Veterinary professionals have to deal with welfare issues in ways that they feel are well-informed, well-reasoned and well-intentioned. So this book provides ways for veterinary professionals to develop their animal welfare understanding, but without them having to become animal welfare research scientists. Science is (as we shall see) vitally important, but veterinary professionals need to be especially aware of the aspects that are important for practice, without trying to recreate the excellent animal welfare literature that already exists. Conversely, I have tried to explain or contextualise the veterinary terms for non-veterinary readers.

Veterinary professionals also want to engage with the bigger picture. So this book also addresses ways in which veterinary professionals can easily, feasibly and realistically contribute to improving animal welfare on a wider scale, through personal efforts and professional bodies. Veterinary professionals can get the best of both worlds by helping both individual patients and making overall progress.

These ideas come from academic research, personal experience and a lot of discussions. As such, I hope it is a contribution to and from all veterinary professionals. I have tended to use *we* and *our* to incorporate all colleagues who work with or within veterinary practice: veterinary surgeons, nurses, scientists, behaviourists, paraprofessionals and lay staff.

The book begins by considering our relationship with our animal patients (Chapter 1), before moving on to consider the other main stakeholders, our clients (Chapter 2). With the main groundwork set out, the chapters can move through the process modelled on how clinical decisions can be made and effected, through animal welfare assessment (Chapter 3), choosing a treatment option (Chapter 4) and achieving the desired goals (Chapter 5). These ideas can then be applied to other animals, people and issues (Chapter 6). Each chapter provides a framework for people to read while considering their own circumstances and concerns.

By no means is this book the work of the sole author. Many people, from many countries, have contributed ideas. Especial thanks to international students, co-lecturers and delegates at undergraduate and postgraduate courses, conferences and seminars around the world, teaching whom has helped me to refine many of the ideas in this book. I would also like to thank those who have discussed drafts of this book. Thanks to practitioners (who mainly advised to make it shorter and include fewer references), especially Nicola Ackerman, Lucy Hamblin, Myfanwy Hill, Richard Hillman, Iain Richards and members of the BVA Ethics and Welfare Group and Council, BSAVA Scientific Committee and SPVS Council. Thanks to animal welfare scientists (who mainly advised to expand points and include more references), especially James Kirkwood, Frank McMillan and Sean Wensley (especially for the last chapter). Thank you to all who gave photographs, as credited, especially Fiona, Jane and Mandy. Thanks also to the anonymous reviewers for useful and positive comments. Finally, belated thanks to many people, but especially David Main, David Morton, Carl Padgett and Peter Sandøe for help and support back when I first started thinking about animal welfare.

Patients

1

1.1 Animal Welfare Accounts

Veterinary professionals are concerned about animal welfare. Animal welfare, loosely defined, is about what is good and bad for animals – what is important for them to achieve and what is important for them to avoid. Veterinary work is about achieving states that are good for animals, such as health and enjoyment of life, and avoiding states that are bad, such as pain and illness. So core aims of veterinary work overlap considerably, if not entirely, with animal welfare concerns. This is why many of us chose to train in veterinary science, medicine or nursing and why most of us wanted to work within the profession.

Every person in the world has an effect on animal welfare. How they treat animals they own or meet; what food and clothes they buy; which charities they give money to; what they enjoy as entertainment and their environmental impact can have an effect on the lives of many animals. This effect may be sometimes beneficial. It may also be harmful. Each person probably effects a combination of harm and benefit (even the kindest people do some harm and even the most evil people may help animals by accident) and has an overall impact on animals' welfare. Each person has an *animal welfare account*, based on all their welfare impacts. If a person does more harm than good, then they have a negative balance. If a person does more good than harm, this is to their *credit*.

Those of us in veterinary practice are especially likely to have significant impacts on the welfare of patients and other animals. Sometimes, we have a positive impact by lessening the harms caused by other people or by natural processes such as

Animal Welfare in Veterinary Practice, First Edition. James Yeates.
© 2013 Universities Federation for Animal Welfare. Published 2013 by Blackwell Publishing Ltd.

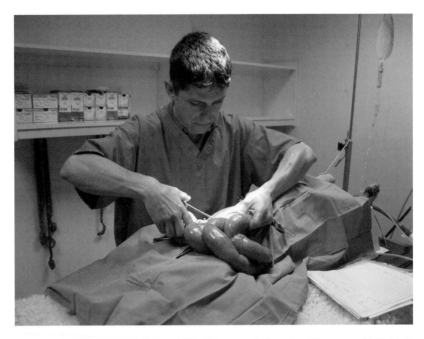

Figure 1.1   Surgery can cause harms as well as provide benefits. (Courtesy of RSPCA Bristol.)

disease. At other times, we have a negative impact by harming animals or helping other people to harm them. Our veterinary roles provide us with *animal welfare capital*, which we can use as an investment to do good but which also gives us opportunities to harm animals – just as borrowing against capital can allow people to incur greater debts. Each of us should make our own animal welfare account as healthy and positive as possible.

Having a healthy animal welfare account requires maximising *welfare credit* and minimising *welfare debt*. Harms should be minimised wherever possible (just as it is not sensible to borrow more than you need). Some harm may be necessary in order to gain bigger welfare benefits, for example when surgery causes pain but cures the animal of a painful condition (which we can think of as an investment). At other times, welfare benefits can be obtained only by taking certain risks, for example where surgery risks causing neuromas or phantom limb pains (Figure 1.1), and we may have to speculate to accumulate.

This approach suggests that we should make every effort to cause good welfare while avoiding causing harms. We could think of this in terms of our overall impact on animal welfare, a sort of *animal welfare footprint*. But it seems better to think of it as each leaving a legacy – good or bad – on animal welfare. Veterinary work provides great opportunities to leave a valuable and significant legacy, and this book may provide some additional suggestions to help readers do even more than they already do.

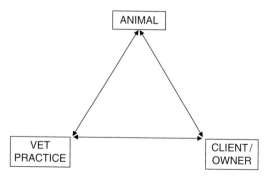

Figure 1.2 Key relationships in veterinary practice.

Whether we consider animal welfare to relate to animals' feelings, their treatment, their biology or their lifestyle, we can be confident that these things are important for animals in some way. This makes veterinary professionals well placed to determine and to achieve animal welfare goals as well. We have an understanding of biological science, interact daily with the pet-owning public and with the animals themselves, and are respected sources of advice in the community. The different people within veterinary practice and professions have different roles and different opportunities to help animals. But we all face similar situations and have the same aims as veterinary professionals.

In this role as veterinary professionals, we face a number of pressures and tensions. We see welfare issues every day, and many are recurrences of seemingly unending problems, despite our good work. We are personally involved in and affected by the pressures, tensions and conflicts we experience. These can cause stress, disillusionment and anger. Some people even leave the veterinary professions, and this is both terribly sad for them and a great loss for animals – especially if it is some of the most welfare-concerned people who are vulnerable to these stresses. We have relationships not only with patients but also with clients (Figure 1.2). In many cases, achieving our animal welfare goals helps people. It can help owners who want their animals' lives, health or behaviour to be improved. It can also help veterinary professionals by reducing the personal and moral stresses and improving profitability. In other cases, we have to balance the conflicting demands. As individual practitioners, we have to balance our wish to achieve our animal welfare goals with client requirements, legal constraints and public concerns. And as professionals, we have to balance being advocates of animal welfare with other goals such as benefitting human society and helping each other. This book looks at how we can best improve animal welfare while respecting these constraints.

We also face conflicts between animals. For example, concern for our patients would lead us to perform caesarians where necessitated by breed conformation. But performing such caesarians perpetuates the problem and allows those conformational traits to continue, leading to increased need for caesarians. In this case, veterinary professionals are both part of the solution and part of the problem. Maintaining a healthy welfare account requires balancing these concerns. In addition, when we do cause harm, either deliberately or through helping our patients, we can improve our welfare account by paying something back. For example, if we perpetuate poor husbandry or breeding (even with the best intentions), then we should *offset* that harm through proactive efforts to promote better practices.

We can maximise our animal welfare account and solve welfare dilemmas by considering many important issues, including the accountability that veterinary professionals have towards animal welfare (discussed in Sections 1.2 and 1.11), our responsibilities (Sections 1.3 and 1.4), the use of science (Section 1.5) and ideas of what is good for animals (Sections 1.6, 1.7, 1.8, 1.9 and 1.10).

1.2 Animal Welfare Accountability

Veterinary professionals have a special role within society that makes their animal welfare accounts especially important and prominent. During the veterinary profession's 250 years, it has become increasingly prominent as a force to improve animal welfare and is increasingly held to account for how it treats animals and how animals are treated by society as a whole. Each veterinary professional has a duty to play their part in helping their profession to fulfil its responsibilities to society.

Modern veterinary practice can be traced back to horse marshals' and farriers' development of medical treatments and surgical procedures, such as firing, bleeding, castrating and tail-docking. By the eighteenth century, such therapies were routinely applied to cattle, sheep and pigs as rising human populations and breeding strategies made individual animals increasingly valuable.

Veterinary practitioners gained a prominent position in safeguarding animal health, but they were far from a profession. This waited upon scientific and medical developments disseminated through education beginning with the first veterinary course in Lyon in the 1760s, followed by others in Alfort, Turin, Copenhagen, Vienna, Dresden, Gottingen, Budapest, Hannover, Padua, Skara and London, and later schools in Toronto, Montreal, Ithaca, Iowa, Santa Catalina, Buenos Aires, Rio de Janeiro and Olinda.

Professional regulation addressed the opportunities for charlatanism (Porter 1992; Hall 1994), with the establishment of professional bodies such as the Royal College of Veterinary Surgeons (RCVS) in 1844, the American Veterinary Medical Association (AVMA) in 1863, the Canadian Veterinary Medical Association (CVMA) in 1949 and the Brazilian "Conselho Federal de Medicina Veterinária" (CFMV) in 1968. These provided society with a guarantee of knowledge, ability and professionalism.

These developments paralleled changes in society at large that increased the respect for animals. Political changes led to widening social progress and protection of vulnerable groups such as slaves, women and children. Scientific discoveries

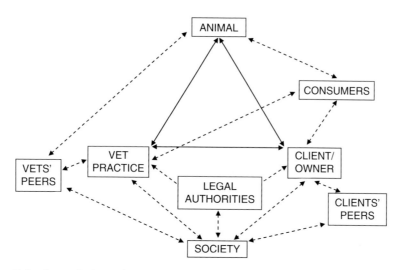

Figure 1.3 Societal relationships in veterinary practice.

highlighted the phenotypic and genetic similarities between humans and other animals. Animals began to gain legal protection, with increasingly progressive laws against specific cruel practices, abuse and vivisection.

By the start of the twentieth century, veterinary professionals had a number of societal responsibilities based not only on their key relationships with owners and patients, but on their wider societal relationships with other animals, governments, other veterinary professionals and society at large (Figure 1.3). Alongside veterinary professionals' primary relationships with animals and clients, the profession also had other vital duties to wider society, such as protecting public health. In addition, the professional status of veterinary practice created new responsibilities for individual practitioners towards their profession and to society.

Since the early twentieth century, there has been a golden age of developments within veterinary science, often paralleling developments in human medicine such as antibiotics, fluid therapy and painkillers and other forms of analgesia. Therapies were often developed on animal experimental subjects, applied to human medical patients, and then adapted to animal medical patients. These developments stimulated the development of veterinary disciplines such as imaging including ultrasound and radiography, immunology to study the bodies' reactions to disease, epidemiology to study the spread of disease, molecular biology to understand the body on a subcellular level, genetics and chemotherapy.

On the one hand, technological developments allowed higher levels of care and, combined with increased treatment of companion animals (Figure 1.4), increased the transference of techniques and protocols from human medicine. On the other hand, technological developments made it feasible to keep animals in high-production systems. Veterinary professionals could prescribe pharmaceuticals,

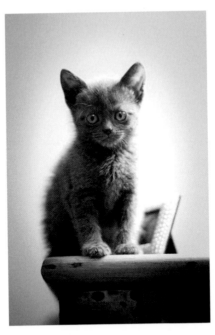

Figure 1.4 The increased importance of companion animals has altered veterinary work. (Courtesy of David Carpenter.)

such as vaccinations and antimicrobials (e.g. penicillins), and operations, such as tail-docking and de-beaking, in order to address system health problems. In some cases, scientific developments went further and advanced methods to increase productivity, such as the use of artificial insemination and growth promoters like bovine somatotropin.

Such changes in modern farming methods prompted a reconsideration of animal welfare issues, which were eloquently and influentially raised by critiques of widespread husbandry practices such as Ruth Harrison in the 1960s and Peter Singer in the 1970s. This led to the creation of animal welfare science as a discipline, promoted especially by the activities of Universities Federation for Animal Welfare (UFAW) since the 1920s, the launch of the Brambell Report in 1965 and the establishment of the UK Farm Animal Welfare Council (FAWC) in 1979. Animal welfare is now an established scientific subject, with its own international journals (e.g. *Animal Welfare*), learned organisations (e.g. UFAW) and academic courses. The development of animal welfare science resulted in a distinction between animal *welfare* and animal *health*. Animals could have their basic physiological and medical needs met despite suffering significant welfare compromises such as frustration, boredom, loneliness and anxiety.

Some people feel the veterinary profession now has a rather poorly defined place in contemporary animal welfare debates due to the implication of practitioners in intensive farming, the veterinary profession's focus on health matters and the separation of health and welfare. Many individual veterinary professionals have contributed considerably to the development of animal welfare science and to policy-making. But they are often a few voices amongst many, and in many countries they lack the authority to provide the determinative viewpoint or the most progressive drive on animal welfare issues. Indeed, in many countries the profession is losing its status as an animal welfare authority.

The risk of losing this status comes while the public, and many veterinary professionals, still appear to consider veterinary professionals' role as being to promote animal welfare. Prominent members of veterinary professions have promised to do more for animal welfare and to concern themselves with wider concerns than only health. Several professional bodies have created structures for individual members to help them advance animal welfare through policy-making, education and specialisation.

The veterinary professions are therefore at a time of both high risk and great opportunity. Our development has provided us with a number of social accountabilities to owners, animals, society and each other. But our historical development can only describe what responsibilities we have had; it cannot prescribe what our responsibilities should be in the future. We have the chance now to decide our core responsibilities and what distinguishes our special place as a profession. Society, many owners and most individual practitioners appear to consider that this focus should be beyond animal health, farming productivity and public health. Society, owners and individual practitioners consider that we should be accountable for animal welfare.

1.3 Animal Welfare Responsibility

If everyone has an *animal welfare account*, then what particular responsibilities do veterinary professionals have? Veterinary professionals have the same general responsibilities to animals as other people but are more accountable because we have more opportunities to cause greater harms and fewer excuses because of our greater knowledge. But veterinary professionals also have duties that laypeople do not.

In many countries, the licence to practise as a veterinary professional is limited to certain people. This restrains other people from conducting potentially harmful procedures. This restriction is beneficial when it stops untrained people from conducting potentially harmful procedures or misusing drugs. But this restriction also places an additional responsibility on those who can provide procedures to do so when necessary, since nobody else can provide them. Such veterinary responsibilities come with our veterinary privileges.

Often veterinary duties are specific responsibilities towards our patients (Yeates 2009a). By taking patients into our care, we are undertaking to work towards maximising their welfare. We have particular duties to those animals, which should motivate us to look after them and provide a certain level of treatment. We have

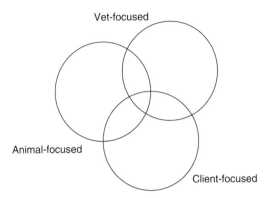

Figure 1.5 Value-based approaches to veterinary decision-making.

duties to owners who have entrusted their animals into the care of veterinary professionals with good faith that those animals will be looked after.

Veterinary professionals have social responsibilities because they have joined a profession where animal welfare concern is expected (Rollin 2006a). Animal welfare responsibilities might be explicitly implied by professional regulations or implicitly required by public expectations. Public expectations include those of society and of other veterinary professionals, whose cooperation and professional relationships are based on that assumption.

Some veterinary professionals specifically promise concern for animal welfare. In the USA, veterinary surgeons may swear the oath of the AVMA, which was recently changed to include a promise "to use my scientific knowledge and skills for the benefit of society through the protection of animal health and welfare, the prevention and relief of animal suffering ..." (AVMA 2011). In Brazil, veterinary surgeons may swear the oath of the CFMV, which includes a promise to "apply my knowledge to scientific and technological development for the benefit of the health and welfare of animals ..." (CFMV 2002). Veterinary professional bodies also often claim to look after animal welfare: by making such a claim, they undertake a responsibility to fulfil it.

Veterinary professionals also have a responsibility to care for animals simply *because* we care about animal welfare. Most applicants for veterinary courses and jobs are highly intelligent and motivated individuals, who could have chosen careers with shorter hours, less stress and better pay. Veterinary professionals have *already* made a choice to sacrifice their personal interests so that they are in a position to help animals. Veterinary surgeons have a responsibility towards animal welfare because they have taken that responsibility on.

Veterinary professionals therefore have a duty to perform *welfare-focused practice*. This approach is an alternative to *vet-focused* practice, which considers the interests of oneself, one's colleagues and one's profession, or *client-focused* practice, which considers the interests of clients, although these three can overlap (Figure 1.5). Veterinary professionals do have duties to clients and themselves, but this book considers that good veterinary practice is predominantly welfare-focused. One is not a good surgeon simply by knowing where to cut. Being a good surgeon involves good decision-making, providing good analgesia and post-operative care and knowing when not to operate. The same animal welfare responsibilities apply in all areas of practice.

1.4 Legal and Professional Responsibilities

Our responsibilities to animal welfare are often underscored by our legal responsibilities. The law provides a backdrop for all our actions, and anxiety about legal consequences can cause unnecessary stress to many veterinary professionals. While this book cannot give legal advice for particular countries, it is possible to sketch certain types of rules that relate how veterinary professionals treat animals alongside the client-focused and owner-focused legal issues discussed in Section 2.2.

Some laws apply to governments and institutions that make decisions. Some countries such as India and Germany include animals in their constitutions. Some international agreements also mandate concern for animals, such as the Treaty of the European Union and the European conventions for the protection of pet animals and animals kept for farming purposes. These laws directly recognise animals' status and prescribe a level of protection. Governments then make laws that apply directly to people, including many elements of criminal law. These laws are interpreted by judicial courts, which make specific decisions about particular cases, with the result that different animals may have inconsistent levels of legal protection.

Many laws proscribe things being done. In most, if not all countries, anti-cruelty legislation is amongst the first pieces of legislation that are brought in. Several countries' laws prevent various negative outcomes, such as causing *unnecessary* suffering, killing animals without good reason, dog fighting or performing certain mutilations. Other laws prescribe positive outcomes, such as caring for an owner's animals, mandating disease control or maintaining biosecurity.

Other laws require things to be done only under certain conditions. For example, many countries' laws state that mutilations such as tail-docking can be performed only on certain animals by certain people using certain methods. Many countries permit experimentation on (vertebrate) animals only under a licence and following ethical review of proposed projects. Several countries require licences for breeding certain animals, owning pet shops, riding schools or boarding kennels or slaughtering an animal for public consumption. Some laws mean people need a licence to own certain animals, such as dangerous animals and farm animals. Often licences are given only under certain conditions, for example that people are trained or have appropriate facilities. More and more countries are requiring licences before people can own any animals at all.

Most countries with an established veterinary profession also have laws that restrict who can practise as veterinary surgeons or veterinary nurses. Often these laws require veterinary professionals to have certain qualifications (e.g. a recognised veterinary degree). Limiting the licence to practise has an additional benefit of allowing the regulation of veterinary professionals. This is often achieved by making membership of the profession conditional upon following certain rules, which are usually described in a deontology or code of practice. These professional rules may prohibit certain welfare-unfriendly procedures, such as kidney transplantation from live donors. They may make other welfare-friendly procedures mandatory, such as emergency first aid. They may also prescribe general approaches such as ensuring the welfare of animals committed to the veterinary professional's care.

Laws and professional rules usually coincide with what society thinks acceptable or unacceptable (e.g. murder). Other laws coordinate action in ways that society thinks useful (e.g. which side of the road to drive on). Often our laws do not tell us what to do but allow a range of options from which we can choose the most acceptable. Consequently, most people follow the law most of the time.

Sometimes the law appears to conflict with what we think is the right thing to do for a particular case. However, this appearance is often misleading. Fortunately, courts often accept a reasonable excuse as a legitimate defence and many prosecutors only proceed when prosecution is in the public interest. For example, a stray animal may be presented in extreme suffering. Thinking only of a law against destruction of property would suggest it should not be given the euthanasia it needs. But the need to avoid unnecessary suffering should provide a legal defence against prosecution for reasonable efforts to prevent suffering. Veterinary professionals should not be *overly* concerned by possible legal ramifications. For example, it may be legitimate to euthanase a stray animal that is suffering only moderately but which is unlikely to be claimed and is unsuitable for rehoming or releasing.

Nevertheless, there may be cases where we might think the law is wrong. Laws may proscribe ways to improve welfare (e.g. stealing someone else's animal) or permit actions that worsen welfare (e.g. shooting or irresponsible breeding). Sometimes following the law may lead to animal welfare compromises, and improving welfare would require breaking the law. Veterinary professionals have a vital role in evaluating the current laws and professional rules and suggesting improvements. This means that welfare-focused decision-making must look beyond simply analysing what our country's law or professional body says.

1.5 Science

Veterinary professionals' education and decisions are prominently based on knowledge generated by the sciences, including animal welfare science and veterinary science. Science is often described as a single way of thinking, but it actually uses several different methods. Hypothetico-deductive approaches start with scientists generating a general hypothesis about the world (e.g. that swans are white). From this, scientists generate more precise and testable hypotheses (e.g. that the next animal of genus *Cygnus* will reflect light of all visual wavelengths). They then obtain data that either support or refute that hypothesis. Inductive methods involve data being collected without any explicit, specific prior hypotheses and analysed to identify relationships such as risk factors. Both methods have advantages and disadvantages and are often combined.

Both hypothetico-deductive and inductive methods are based on a number of features that make them *scientific*. Both use relatively simple observations that are consistent between people, quantitative data analysed using standardised statistical methods based on agreed mathematical axioms. In this way, both use *building blocks* to work from simple agreed ideas to more complex conclusions, with which people should agree, using which should be repeatable in different situations and at different times.

These efforts to make science more reliable mean that science is seen as a way to obtain objective knowledge. Non-scientific beliefs can be inaccurate because they involve an invalid generalisation or because they are skewed. Beliefs involve an invalid generalisation when they are based on a limited number of observations, which relate only to specific, non-representative animals. Such beliefs can include those based on an owner's personal experiences of their previous animals or a veterinary professional's personal experiences of their previous cases. Beliefs may be skewed when they are influenced by individual biases, which alter a person's interpretation of the observations. These include *confirmation biases*, where we tend to take more notice of observations that confirm what we already believe, *self-interest biases*, where we tend to be more ready to believe facts that we want to be true, and *emotional biases*, where our beliefs are affected by our emotions.

The objectivity of science makes it a valuable tool in decision-making, especially in determining trustworthy factual beliefs. Veterinary professionals should encourage the use of science in decision-making, both within evidence-based veterinary medicine and within veterinary and animal welfare policy-making, and it is good for decisions to be based on science. However, decisions should not – indeed cannot – be based *only* on science, for several reasons. Science also has its limitations, just like law.

In many cases, there simply is no scientific information. Some subjects are not studied because the results are obvious without the need for the study, some because they are not sufficiently interesting to scientists or funders, and some because they concern hypotheses or things that would be unethical to test. For example, it would seem wrong to study the effects of chainsaw injuries on cows. So we do not have any scientific data on bovine chainsaw injuries. Nevertheless, we can have a fairly confident belief that chainsaws will cause tissue damage, haemorrhage and pain behaviours, based on our personal experience of similar injuries and common sense. Such absences of data mean we cannot say that decisions should be made only when scientific data are available, although this position is expressed quite often by people trying to preserve the status quo. In many cases, we can – and should – make decisions about how confident we are that a treatment will work, often based on experience or understanding of physiology, pathology and pharmacology or simple common sense.

Even where scientific data are produced, studies are not always 100% accurate. Studies can involve errors, chance effects, subconscious biases (e.g. in interpreting data) or even conscious manipulation (e.g. publication biases). Studies may therefore disagree, and we have to choose which data we use, and this choice is often a non-scientific choice. This means it can be skewed or biased, and this is especially dangerous if the final decision is then presented as completely scientific. There is also a danger that people dress up facts to look more scientific, for example by presenting them pseudo-scientifically as numbers or as surveys. So, even where data are available, we must use science appropriately and critically.

Even where there are reliable scientific data, there can be limits to what those data can prove. Results can demonstrate statistical probabilities about the animals that were studied in the experiment or study (often compared to pure chance, e.g. in "p" values). However, these probabilities may not apply to other animals in other situations (e.g. other species or individuals). Decisions whether to extrapolate are yet more non-scientific decisions about whether that extrapolation is justified.

Furthermore, there are some things that science cannot prove because they are outside of scientific methodologies. Three examples are especially important for us: death, feelings and the future. If animal welfare science assesses what happens to an animal (while it exists), then it cannot study what does not happen to the animal while it no longer exists. If science assesses observable events, and animals' feelings are unobservable, then science cannot prove that animals have feelings. If science describes what occurs in the past, then it cannot describe what will occur in the future.

Veterinary professionals therefore need to use other methods to convert scientific information into animal welfare assessments and decisions. This inevitably – and beneficially – involves using both emotional processing and logical, comprehensive and critical reasoning. Fortunately, these are skills that veterinary professionals develop. We have an understanding of the limitations of science, an appreciation of probability and uncertainty, an ability to tailor evidence to individual cases and experience to make future assessments. These are all valuable skills that go beyond science that veterinary professionals can possess.

1.6 Achieving and Avoiding

Veterinary professionals have the skills to use information, reasoning and judgement to work out what is worth achieving or avoiding. These decisions are an essential part of animal welfare assessment and clinical decision-making.

Many things are worth achieving or avoiding for other humans. We often think we should help, or at least not harm, our clients, such as by giving them value for

---

Box 1.1   Examples of what may be important for animals.

Negative feelings (e.g. pain)
Positive feelings (e.g. pleasure)
Satisfaction of negative preferences (avoiding what it wants to avoid)
Satisfaction of positive preferences (achieving what it wants)
Health or biological functioning
Longevity
Productivity (e.g. milk production or feed conversion ratio)
Naturalness of behaviours (similarity to wild equivalents)
Normalness of behaviour relative to itself at other times
Normalness of behaviour relative to similar animals in similar circumstances
Naturalness of environment
Freedom
Quality of care and husbandry
Intentions of carer (e.g. cruelty versus neglect)

---

money. We often think we should help, or at least not harm, other humans, such as by minimising public health risks. Treating animals can provide worthwhile human benefits such as companionship, financial profit, experimental data and food, alongside human harms such as emotional stress, financial costs, aggression and zoonotic diseases that humans can catch from non-human animals.

Some things are worth achieving or avoiding for ourselves. We may think we should develop our expertise and knowledge, make money, satisfy intellectual curiosity and avoid guilt, grief, regret or litigation. Treating animals can provide worthwhile benefits to oneself, such as respect, financial profit, experimental data and education, or harms to oneself, such as emotional stress, financial costs, zoonotic diseases and aggression.

Other things are worth achieving or avoiding for the animals. There are many things that veterinary professionals or owners may think are worth achieving for animals (Box 1.1). Many of these things have *indirect* value for animals. Things with indirect value are worth achieving or worth avoiding for an explicable reason – you can answer the question "Why is that good/bad?" with an explanation. Some such factors *cause* an animal's welfare to improve or worsen. These can be described as *welfare inputs* (Figure 1.6). Some important factors that influence animals' welfare include the five welfare needs listed in Box 1.2. Other factors that cause good or bad welfare are even more removed, such as veterinary professionals receiving quality training, which should lead to better welfare for animals they treat. Other indirectly valuable things may *signify* that an animal's welfare has improved or worsened. These can be described as *welfare symptoms*. Such welfare symptoms are things that are caused by feelings (e.g. a pain response) or that are caused by things that also cause feelings (a symptom of a developing disease), as

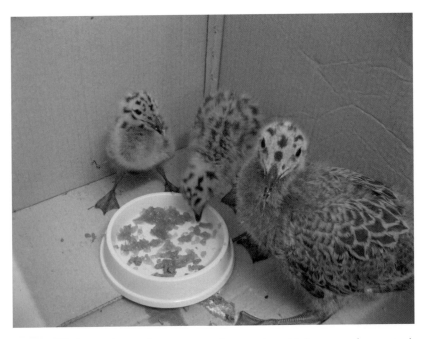

Figure 1.6 Food has indirect value as an *input* because it avoids hunger and promotes health. (Courtesy of RSPCA Bristol.)

Box 1.2   Five welfare needs (adapted from Animal Welfare Act 2006).

- Need for a suitable environment
- Need for a suitable diet
- Need to be able to exhibit normal behaviour patterns
- Need for the company of, or to be apart from, other animals
- Need to be protected against pain, suffering, injury and disease

---

represented in Figure 1.7. In some cases, signs of welfare problems are more removed from the animal, such as a line on a radiograph that indicates a fracture. Welfare inputs and symptoms of welfare are not always good or bad for animals in themselves. Veterinary training is not good for animals if the veterinary professional becomes an estate agent. A line on an x-ray is not bad if it turns out to be an artefact from the developer.

Causes and symptoms can be used to work out what is worth achieving or avoiding *directly*. For example, veterinary care is good for animals not in itself but because it helps to prevent or cure problems such as disease (and we would probably not mind a world without veterinary treatment if there was no need for that treatment). Disease is bad for animals because it causes them to suffer feelings of

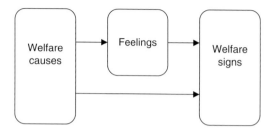

Figure 1.7 Causes and signs of good or bad animal welfare.

illness, such as pain and malaise (and we tend to be unconcerned by completely benign conditions). Feelings such as pain and malaise are bad in themselves. We can explain such feelings in terms of evolutionary or sociobiology, as drivers for appropriate behaviour, but we would still think they were worth avoiding regardless of their effects or their implications – such feelings are directly important. Similarly, health is good because it prevents suffering. Food is good because it is enjoyable and prevents hunger. For many veterinary professionals, thinking through such chains of questioning often end with statements about animals' feelings, leading to the conclusion that what have direct value for animals are the feelings that they experience.

This book deliberately does not define animal welfare or quality-of-life too narrowly. Many people have tried to define animal welfare, and the term is often used to mean whatever people want it to mean (Webster 2005). In fact, we do not need a rigid definition for animal welfare any more than we need a definitive meaning of veterinary, or even health. This book considers animal welfare as a vague idea of what is in animals' interests, i.e. what is directly good or bad for them as individuals. Feelings are central to this idea, but veterinary professionals should also consider things that can cause and signify feelings as well.

1.7 Feelings

Not every feeling is directly important. There is nothing intrinsically good or bad about the experience of recognition or the experience of seeing something yellow (or ultraviolet). What makes a feeling good or bad is whether it is pleasant or unpleasant – its *valence*. Pleasant feelings, with a positive valence, are intrinsically good; unpleasant feelings, with a negative valence, are intrinsically bad. An animal's welfare is good if its pleasant feelings outweigh its unpleasant feelings. An input is good for an animal's welfare if it makes the animal experience pleasant feelings or prevents it from experiencing unpleasant feelings.

A list of unpleasant and pleasant feelings is given in Table 1.1, with no attempt to separate those that different species have and do not have. Most are feelings with which veterinary professionals are familiar, but some features are worth elaborating.

Table 1.1 Feelings some animals may experience.

Positive feelings	Negative feelings
Anticipation	Fear
Comfort	Discomfort
Confidence	Doubt
Contentment	Restlessness
Control	Confusion
	Frustration
	Helplessness
	Resignation
Curiosity	Ennui
Interest	
Euphoria	Dysphoria
Excitement	Boredom
Expectation	Anxiety
Fellow-feeling	Loneliness
	Xenophobia
Gustatory pleasure	Disgust
Lust	
Maternal–infant affection	
Playfulness	
Relaxedness	Fatigue
Relief	Disappointment
Satiety	Hunger
	Over-fullness
Satisfaction	Distress
Sexual pleasure	
	Shock
Tactile pleasure	Pain
	Pruritus (itchiness)
	Thirst
Trust	Mistrust
Vitality	Illness
	Malaise
Wanting to achieve something	Wanting to avoid something
Ambivalence	

Many feelings have both negative and positive opposites (although not all, e.g. there is no positive correlate to thirst). For example, the pleasant feeling of general elation or well-being described as *euphoria* is opposite to an unpleasant feeling of general unease or disquiet often described as *dysphoria*. Similarly, some gregarious animals may experience a pleasant emotion which may be described as *fellow-feeling* when they are part of a collective group, such as their herd, flock,

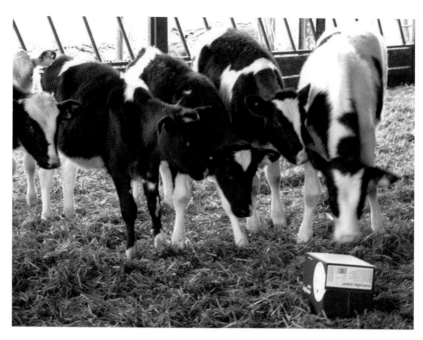

Figure 1.8 Fear and curiosity both involve high arousal but are of different valence. (Courtesy of James Yeates.)

pack or shoal – and veterinary professionals may feel this as part of their profession. This fellow-feeling has two opposites. One is loneliness, which gregarious animals like cows, sheep, pigs, dogs, horses and rabbits may experience when isolated. Another is *xenophobia*, which non-gregarious animals like cats and hamsters may experience when in unwelcome company (alongside other feelings such as fear). As another example, a lack of stimulation can lead to *boredom, ennui* or even *apathy* (a lack of feelings). Boredom has several opposites, such as *interest* and *flow*, which is the feeling one gets when thoroughly engaged in a task (Csikszentmihalyi 1999).

Feelings can vary not only in terms of valence but also in *arousal*, which is the animal's level of excitation or activation (Figure 1.8). Feelings may be high arousal and negative valence (e.g. fear), high arousal and positive valence (e.g. excitement), low arousal and positive valence (e.g. contentment) or low arousal and negative valence (e.g. boredom). As these examples show, arousal is not obviously good or bad in itself. (Recent work also suggests another way feelings can vary in terms of the animal's level of *control, dominance* or *potency*.)

Some feelings relate to animals' motivations, such as *desire, anticipation* and *lust*. Some are caused by such motivations being fulfilled or not, such as *frustration* and *satisfaction*. Other feelings involve the affective experience based on what animals have already, such as *liking* and *pain*. In many cases, animals will experience both motivational and affective feelings, for example if they are experiencing pain they will also be motivated to end that pain.

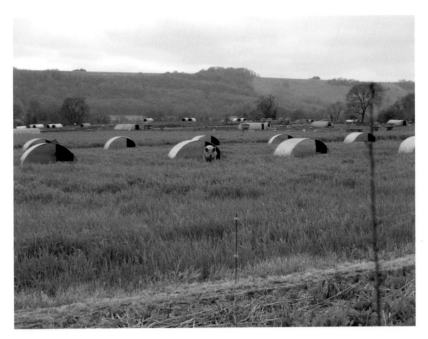

Figure 1.9 Domestic pigs may suffer similar or different feelings to wild pigs or to humans. (Courtesy of James Yeates.)

Another relevant difference is between more transient emotions versus more persistent moods, such as happiness, sadness, confidence and depression. Such moods may affect an animal's personality, temperament and behaviour, allowing us to describe them as *sociable*, *playful* or *withdrawn* and as *optimistic* or *pessimistic* in terms of how they interpret ambiguous stimuli and risks.

Feelings may also be differentiated into *basic* and *higher* feelings, depending on the amount of cortical processing required. *Basic* emotions appear to involve relatively little processing and correlate largely to midbrain and limbic structures. These include feelings of pain, fear, lust, pleasure, etc. *Higher* feelings involve more processing in the brain cortices, especially in prefrontal cortical regions. These include feelings of guilt, shame, embarrassment, spite, pride and existential angst. The evidence that non-human animals experience such *higher* emotions is unclear, although there is growing evidence that some animals can have feelings such as injustice, doubt and grief.

One final important distinction between different feelings is in terms of which animals experience which feelings. Different species may experience different feelings, depending on their underlying biology and neurology, and the ecological niches and social contexts in which they have evolved. Indeed, the same feelings may not be experienced by animals of different breeds or genders or by those in different habitats. As an example in humans, the emotion of *being like a wild pig*, where people run amok, may be experienced only by New Guinean men – and perhaps wild pigs (Figure 1.9). Similarly, some feelings such as maternal affection

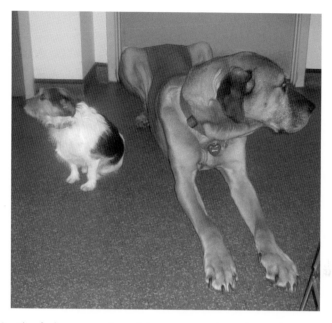

Figure 1.10 The feelings experienced in company depends on the species and on the individual. (Courtesy of RSPCA Bristol.)

may be experienced only by females in many species where only the females are involved in caring for their young. In addition, different *individuals* may experience different emotions, even in the same situations, For example, the aforementioned species-based attribution of *fellow-feeling, loneliness* and *xenophobia* is over-simplistic: individuals in gregarious species may have different relationships with different individual conspecifics (Figure 1.10). It is vital for veterinary professionals to recognise possible human–animal differences, differences between non-human animal species and differences between individuals. At the same time, it seems highly likely that many emotions, especially *basic* emotions such as fear and pain, are experienced by most individuals of most domestic species.

1.8 Inferring Feelings

If feelings are worth achieving or avoiding, then the problem that science cannot observe feelings becomes a significant issue for veterinary professionals. We can see directly into our own minds (which was the observation that allowed René Descartes to conclude that he existed), but we cannot directly observe the feelings of other animals or of other humans (Figure 1.11).

Faced with this *problem of other minds*, some people give up. Positivist scientists argued that science should not study animals' emotions and that we should not be concerned with animals' feelings in deciding what to do. Fortunately, most

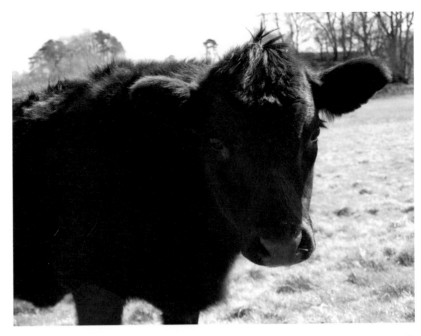

Figure 1.11 We cannot directly observe other animals' subjective feelings. (Courtesy of James Yeates.)

veterinary professionals use our common sense, which suggests that other animals and humans probably do have feelings. This common-sense approach is especially fortunate given that people cannot observe each others' emotions, but few scientists argued that other people should ignore scientists' welfare.

So how can we read other minds? Effectively, we must infer animals' feelings by comparing oneself ("I") and other animals ("them"). As an individual, I look at my feelings in certain situations and then compare other animals to myself. Where there are similarities, I infer that those animals have similar feelings. We can then compare other animals and humans with each other.

In practice, we tend to compare three things about ourselves and animals: their *context* (i.e. what is happening to them), their *biology* (especially their neurobiology) and their *responses* (e.g. their behaviour). If a vertebrate animal has an injury of a kind that would cause me pain (e.g. a skin burn), has similar biology to me (e.g. inflammatory processes, ascending nerves that carry impulses from damaged tissues and a central nervous system) and acts like I would act if I were in pain (e.g. withdrawing or vocalising), then I may infer that this animal is feeling pain. Such comparisons give us ideas of what things have indirect value because they cause or signify feelings, as in Table 1.2.

This approach is sometimes called *anthropomorphism*, but since the basic comparison is with oneself, rather than between animals and humans in general, a

Table 1.2 Comparative assessments used for causes and symptoms of feelings.

	Cause of feelings	**Signs of feelings**
Type of comparison used	Context-based	Behaviour-based
What to assess	Inputs	Symptoms

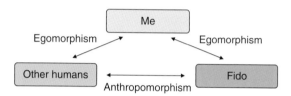

Figure 1.12 Inferring other's feelings can involve *egomorphism* (comparing to oneself) and *anthropomorphism* (comparing to humans).

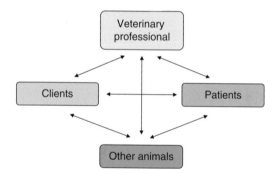

Figure 1.13 Comparisons for inferring mental states between humans and animals.

better term is *egomorphism* (Figure 1.12). It is easier to *egomorphise* with other humans, since they are more similar to me, but one can also make comparisons with other animals. One can also make comparison from other humans to other animals (which is more accurately described as *anthropomorphism*), from some animals to others (the basis of many animal welfare and veterinary scientific experiments) and from animals to humans (the basis of many experiments in biomedical sciences). Figure 1.13 shows the different relevant comparisons in veterinary practice.

The use of relevant comparisons should also bear in mind relevant *differences*. I am different to other humans and experience different feelings in different situations. Similarly, I am different to other animals and so may expect we will experience different feelings in different situations. Recognition of differences

---

Box 1.3   Inferred deep similarities between oneself and other animals.

- Animals have feelings
- Animals' feelings can change with time and circumstances
- Animals' feelings can relate to their contexts (contexts cause feelings)
- Animals' responses can relate to their feelings (responses indicate feelings)
- Animals feelings often correlate with biological responses (e.g. cortisol)
- Animals often do what they are motivated to do (behaviours indicate motivations)
- Animals are often motivated to do what they enjoy (motivational feelings coincide with affective feelings)
- Animals may experience negative feelings when their motivations are frustrated
- Animals can learn, based on feelings (e.g. conditioning)

---

means that veterinary professionals must not unthinkingly conclude that other animals experience the same feelings as humans. By the same token, differences also mean that we should recognise that other humans – including owners and colleagues – may experience very different emotions in circumstances and react very differently. This recognition of differences is part of *critical anthropomorphism* (or *critical egomorphism*).

It is easy to say that we should consider similarities and differences, but it is harder to work out when we should infer that animals experience similar feelings versus when we should infer they experience different feelings. The best way to do this is to look at deeper comparisons of more basic similarities, which can then give us generic descriptions by which to evaluate more superficial similarities and differences. For example, we can infer very basic similarities such as those in Box 1.3. (Sometimes these comparisons are so deep or general we do not even notice they are comparisons.) From these comparisons we can identify relevant differences.

Here are two simple examples. I enjoy eating chips. I could unthinkingly infer that cows also enjoy chips. Cows and I are similar in lots of ways (we both have stomachs, teeth and nipples, we both salivate, chew, digest, walk and vocalise, etc.). Cows and I are also different in lots of ways (they are heavier, wear less clothes, ruminate, have more stomachs, produce more milk, etc.), and some of these differences may be relevant. I can try to determine which differences are relevant by identifying deep similarities. I can observe that both cows and I are motivated to eat certain foodstuffs, that cows and I salivate on smelling certain foods, that cows and I have certain foods that appear suited to their gut biology and flora and so on. I infer a deep similarity: that we both enjoy those foods that we are motivated to eat, salivate on smelling and can digest. I observe that, for cows, these apply not to chips but to, say, total mixed rations (TMR) or grass. I infer that cows enjoy eating TMR or grass. As another example, I am scared of neither veterinary practices nor fireworks. But I tremble, show physiological stress responses and avoid things that do scare me, and I infer the same for dogs. So when a dog trembles during firework displays or resists entering a practice, I infer it is scared.

Another deep similarity between animals and humans is that both our feelings appear to have evolved over time to help us respond to our environments. Feelings like pleasure and pain allow conditioning-based learning. Feelings like fear allow rapid *fight, flight or freeze* responses. Because feelings have evolved to help animals respond to their environments, they are likely to be caused by their environment and health (Boissy *et al.* 2007a) and to lead to (i.e. be indicated by) physiological changes and behaviours (Denton *et al.* 2009). This means that we can relate animals' feelings to their environment at the time and the environment in which they evolved.

Such reasoning allows us to identify a number of causes and symptoms of animals' feelings. Scientific studies and personal experience can add evidence to support a hypothesis that animals feel a certain feeling in a certain context, although this evidence is always circumstantial. More experience, agreement and scientific data can make us more confident that an animal will experience a certain emotion in a certain circumstance and that this circumstance is therefore worth achieving or avoiding. Some symptoms are also causes. Self-harming can both indicate pain and cause it. Chronic stress responses can lead to diseases such as gastric ulceration.

1.9 Pathological Causes of Feelings

Pathological causes of feelings, and their symptoms, are central to traditional veterinary practice. This section therefore cannot describe the myriad different pathological states and processes that animals suffer, so readers are referred to further reading. Instead, this section will concentrate on the issue of what pathological states mean in terms of welfare.

Some early animal welfare scientists thought of health as being directly important for animals. This facilitated the scientific investigation of animal welfare, because disease states and injuries can be readily observed and often quantified, and maintained a link between animal welfare and veterinary science. However, health does not have direct importance insofar as we can say that health and disease are worth achieving and avoiding because they relate to animals' feelings.

Health compromises are certainly important causes of feelings. Diseases and injuries may cause feelings of *illness*, such as nausea, pruritus, fatigue and malaise (Figure 1.14). Conversely, health may cause a feeling of *vitality* or *vigour*. This means that helping animals to get or stay healthy is a major part of improving their welfare. Prophylactic treatments can prevent problems. Remedial treatments can cure conditions. Palliative treatments can reduce the feelings caused by the condition without curing the condition. Palliating the feelings caused by disease and injury will also minimise welfare harms. Veterinary professionals therefore have a major role in improving animals' welfare.

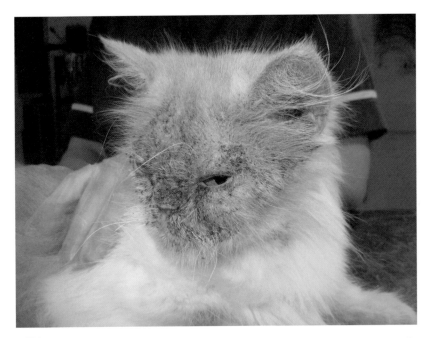

Figure 1.14 Disease can cause animals to experience unpleasant feelings like discomfort and pain. (Courtesy of RSPCA Bristol.)

Health is also important as a sign of welfare problems. Increased susceptibility to disease can suggest chronic stress. Self-mutilation or psychological conditions can signify underlying mental stress. Speed of recovery from illness may also indicate animals' welfare, with negative feelings slowing healing and positive feelings enhancing recovery, as suggested by research in humans (Pressman & Cohen 2005), mice (Hockly *et al.* 2002) and rats (Passineau *et al.* 2001).

Mental health is one element of health with clear links to feelings. Many psychological or behavioural disorders can be associated with underlying motivational or affective feelings. Some veterinary professionals think of mental health as being part of a health-based concept of welfare. This is slightly misleading. Good mental health is not the same as happiness. Some animals (or people) may be completely sane but still unhappy; others may be completely insane but happy. Mental health is a useful concept for veterinary professionals, but one still needs to consider whether good or bad mental health causes pleasant or unpleasant feelings.

Poor health is additionally important as a deprivation. When an animal has a disability, it may not be able to do things that it enjoys. Such disability may cause frustration if the animal remains motivated to perform that action, such as a pig with a nose-ring, a horse with an anti-windsucking collar, a de-vocalised dog or a de-clawed cat. Deprivations can also be considered harmful to an animal even if an animal does not consciously *miss* anything, because the animal would be better off with whatever it lacks (just as if someone defrauded me of an inheritance without me ever knowing about it).

One specific way in which poor health deprives animals of feelings is when it causes death. The process of dying is a cause of welfare harms insofar as the process of *dying* can cause negative feelings such as pain, malaise or fear.

Being dead prevents an animal having any feelings at all. Indeed, if an animal does not exist, then sentences like "this animal suffers..." make no sense. This means that being dead is not *directly* important for animals, hence the idea that "death is not a welfare issue" (Webster 1994). More specifically, being dead causes an animal to avoid the feelings it would have had if it had lived (Yeates 2009b). When the avoided feelings are pleasant, then they are worth achieving, and being dead deprives the animal of those feelings. When the avoided feelings are unpleasant, then they are worth avoiding, so being dead is beneficial. So death is indirectly important for animals. In fact, we can say that life is also not directly important to animals – life is important insofar as it causes feelings. A life that involves mainly pleasure is worth achieving. A life that involves considerable suffering is not worth achieving; rather it is worth being avoided.

Death can also function as a sign of animals' welfare. More accurately, the *time* of death can be an indicator of an animal's welfare throughout its life. A decreased longevity suggests that the animal had higher risks, greater demands or more stress during its life. By the same logic, one can also use the mortality rate within a herd or a treatment group in a clinical trial as an indicator of the group's overall welfare. However, longevity and mortality rates are not accurate indicators. There may be significant inter-individual variation, which would need to be compensated for by averaging over many animals. In addition, many welfare problems are not fatal and so will not decrease longevity or increase mortality rates. Indeed, when suffering animals are kept alive by veterinary treatment, then increased survival time actually indicates worse welfare. This highlights the fact that veterinary treatment can lead to significant welfare compromises, and this is worth considering in more detail.

1.10 Iatrogenic Causes of Feelings

While veterinary professionals can help improve welfare by preventing, curing or palliating pathological causes of feelings, they also risk worsening welfare. Some of these risks are from misuse or errors, but some risks occur when therapies are used appropriately. These can be called *iatrogenic* harms in that they are caused by veterinary treatment (Yeates 2012a).

Iatrogenic harms are a risk not only in cases such as cosmetic mutilations (e.g. ear-cropping), which have limited welfare benefits, but in all veterinary interventions. Iatrogenic harms are part of each veterinary professional's welfare account. Every treatment involves a *welfare gamble* that the benefits will outweigh the harms, and veterinary professionals should try to make only rational and safe bets.

The most obvious welfare harm is pain. Operations or other interventions can involve tissue damage and inflammation. Animals may show post-operative pain-related behaviours, either local to the affected area (e.g. hypersensitivity, allodynia, lameness, licking and self-mutilation) or more general (e.g. inactivity or increased activity, hyperalgesia and altered moods) and physiological responses (e.g. increased heart rate, respiratory rate, blood glucose or cortisol levels, altered immune function, C-reactive protein and haptoglobin levels). From such causes and signs, we may infer that animals can experience post-operative pain.

Treatments can cause other feelings of illness. Vaccines and cancer chemotherapeutics may induce malaise. Anaesthesia and analgesia can cause dysphoria. Medications can cause adverse drug reactions. Surgery, joint treatments, cerebrospinal fluid sampling or blood sampling can cause infections, tissue reactions or thrombosis, with the subsequent clots causing tissue damage. Certain surgeries can increase the risk of specific harms, for example neutering is associated with predispositions to obesity and total ear canal removal (TECA) with facial nerve damage (as well as deafness).

Some therapies can cause fear. Dealing with problem behaviours symptomatically, without addressing underlying anxieties, can worsen problems. Classically, prescribing acepromazine for noise phobias may increase fear (Overall 1997; Sherman & Mills 2008), and symptomatic anti-vice treatments may increase horses' stress (McBride & Cudderford 2001). More generally, veterinary treatment can cause fear through catching and transporting (Figure 1.15) and handling animals (Figure 1.16). Veterinary contact may be especially stressful if animals are rarely handled, such as wild or feral animals and some farm or exotic species, but even pet dogs may be nervous of humans (Rooney *et al.* 2007; Siracusa *et al.* 2008). Many domestic animals demonstrate what might be called *vet-fear*. Vet-fear varies between different animal individuals, for example some dogs may specifically fear males (Hennessy *et al.* 1997; Wells & Hepper 1999) or one particular clinician (Timmins *et al.* 2007).

Hospitalisation or isolation can cause distress, whether on the farm or yard or in a practice. A lack of space can lead to lack of exercise and boredom. Lack of conspecific (or human) company can cause *isolation stress*. Animals suffer a disruption of their normal routine and an inability to predict or control their environment (e.g. hospitalised dogs cannot choose when to go to the toilet). Consequently, isolated animals often show behaviours that may indicate welfare problems, such as vocalisations, repetitive behaviours and hyperactivity or lethargy.

Veterinary professionals may also perpetuate existing welfare problems. Life-saving treatment of suffering animals perpetuates that suffering. More subtly, suggesting or providing treatment gives owners an opportunity not to opt for euthanasia, a glimmer of hope that their animal may get better if it is not killed and a legitimacy to

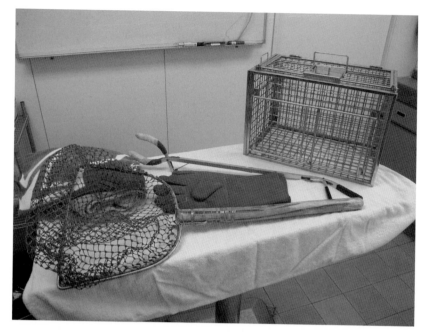

Figure 1.15 Catching can cause iatrogenic harm to animals, so it needs to be done as humanely as possible. (Courtesy of SPCA Hong Kong.)

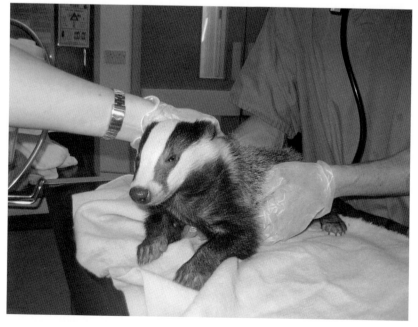

Figure 1.16 Handling can cause fear, especially for wild animals. (Courtesy of RSPCA Bristol.)

perpetuating its life despite its suffering. This can create a dilemma for veterinary professionals who want to offer palliation without perpetuating animals' suffering.

Veterinary professionals may also cause or facilitate further welfare problems to our patients. Providing pain relief to keep overworked horses in work allows that overwork to continue. Fracture repair or neurectomies may increase racehorses' risk of injury because the repair causes subsequent weakness or the removal of part of a nerve causes a loss of feeling. For example, the use of drugs such as antimicrobials (e.g. coccidiostats) or mutilations (e.g. tail-docking) may allow animals to be kept in unsuitable conditions such as impoverished pig systems.

Veterinary professionals can also cause iatrogenic harms to *other* animals. Hospitalising an animal with an infectious condition can lead to other animals contracting nosocomial infections in the hospital. Similarly, saving an animal with an infectious condition can lead to other animals catching that disease. Misuse of antibiotics or antiparasitics may lead to resistance that make these drugs ineffective for other patients.

Veterinary professionals can even cause harms to *future* animals. In some cases, treatments for breed-related conditions may perpetuate those conditions within the breed. For example, repairing genetic defects such as hernias without also neutering the animal may hide those defects and lead to their being passed on. Similarly, performing caesarians can propagate dystocias. In other cases, providing treatment to address some of the problems caused by welfare-unfriendly husbandry systems (e.g. widespread coccidiostats) may paradoxically perpetuate those husbandry systems by making them feasible. Treating breed-related conditions makes those breeds less of a bad purchase, since owners can purchase animals that will suffer future problems (e.g. atopy) but then treat those conditions (to some degree).

1.11 Beyond Health

Pathological and iatrogenic causes of animal welfare are not the only things that affect animals' lives. There are many other elements which are discussed in the next chapter. However, it is worth describing why these other causes should be important to veterinary professionals. There is an argument that veterinary professionals should be concerned only about health-related issues. There are several arguments in response to this.

A prophylactic argument is that many other aspects of welfare relate to health. So dealing only with health will still involve dealing with lots of other welfare issues indirectly. Since welfare problems can lead to health problems, preventative medicine should involve tackling those underlying welfare issues.

A clinical argument is that veterinary professionals should be concerned about welfare because mental states can affect healing and recovery. Thus, clinical success on rectifying health problems may be enhanced by addressing other elements of patients' welfare at the same time.

A responsibility-based argument is that veterinary professionals should be concerned about those welfare problems that they cause. This includes iatrogenic harms in the surgery, and the duty to avoid causing welfare problems underlies the medical doctrine of "first, do no harm". This concern should extend to mitigating the effect of clinical advice, and veterinary professionals should at least be aware of where their recommendations may lead to compromises.

An expertise-based argument is that veterinary professionals have the knowledge, practicality and decision-making ability to make the best decisions, or at least to contribute valuably. If veterinary professionals tackle only health-related welfare issues, then who should tackle other welfare problems – "If not you, then who"? No other profession has the general knowledge, experience, practicality or respect, so veterinary professionals cannot pass the buck.

An autonomy-based argument is that leaving the public animal welfare agenda to non-veterinary groups, the resultant decisions will impact on veterinary practice whether we like it or not. It seems better for the profession to be involved in setting, and implementing, that agenda.

A definitional argument is that health involves or requires some degree of good welfare by definition. At the very least, health should include mental health. While mental health does not map perfectly onto welfare, nevertheless many welfare issues relate to poor mental health.

An undertaking-based argument is that veterinary professionals in many countries have *claimed* to address welfare issues. This may be a defensive tactic to prevent other people having more influence, in which case the claim is hypocritical. It may be an aspiration to be fulfilled, in which case there is a need to fulfil it. Either way, there is a grave danger if a respected profession fails to deliver on a promise to effectively advocate for animals. This danger is to animals, who will not be fully represented, and to the profession, who will seem arrogant and conspicuously uncaring.

A commercial argument is that veterinary professionals stand to gain from being at the forefront on welfare issues. People usually want their animal to be happier and are often willing to pay for it. Individual practices could therefore market themselves directly as helping animals' welfare. Indeed, the profession itself stands to gain from being seen as animal advocates. Happier animals should mean happier clients. Happier clients can be more willing to pay.

A legal argument is that the animal welfare laws of many countries apply to veterinary professionals as to owners. Most prosecuting bodies appear reluctant to prosecute veterinary professionals for welfare offences, but this may not always be the case. Veterinary professionals, at least in many countries, do have a legal duty to care for their animals.

A prudential argument is that veterinary surgeons often end up with the unpleasant job of rectifying problems caused by poor welfare, not least the killing of unwanted or unrehomable animals. Many of these problems do not earn the practice much money, but they are emotionally draining, lead to stress and poor work relationships and decrease job satisfaction. It seems sensible for veterinary professionals to try to prevent such situations from occurring.

A more positive argument is that veterinary professionals can enjoy helping animals. This is, after all, why many became veterinary professionals. Making a difference can feel better than making a profit. Driving animal welfare improvements in the wider world can feel good too.

Summary and key recommendations

- Everyone has an animal welfare account to maximise. Veterinary professionals have particular responsibilities towards animal welfare due to their knowledge, abilities, legal privilege and personal undertakings. Most veterinary professionals are concerned about animal welfare and are well placed to help but face a number of pressures and obstacles. This makes us part of the solution and part of the problem.
- Animal welfare *science* uses hypothetico-deductive and inductive approaches. Neither the law nor science can always tell us what to do. Decisions need to be based not only on science but also on emotions and values. Veterinary professionals are experts at applying science to individual cases.
- Pleasant (positively valenced) feelings are worth achieving. Unpleasant (negatively valenced) feelings are worth avoiding. Things may have value because they *cause* or *signify* better or worse feelings. Science cannot prove or disprove animals' feelings. We can egomorphically compare animal's and our own context, biology and responses. We must consider relevant me–other differences, by considering deeper similarities.
- Pathologies are important causes of unpleasant feelings. Death avoids good and bad feelings. Veterinary professionals have a duty to consider other causes of feelings. Veterinary professionals can cause iatrogenic harms or perpetuate welfare problems for non-patient animals.

Selected further reading

Further information on the history of the veterinary profession is provided by Dunlop and Williams (1996), Hatschbach (2006) and Swabe (1999), and the specific implications of the increased small animal work are discussed by Brown and Silverman (1999).

Further historical information on animal welfare movement is provided by Fraser (2007). Overviews of animal welfare concepts are provided by Nordenfelt (2006), Broom (2008), Webster (2005) and Can be found in FAWC (2009). The idea of direct welfare importance is discussed by Yeates (2010a). The significance of the negative versus positive, valence versus arousal and affect versus motivation divides are discussed by Yeates and Main (2008).

There are hundreds of veterinary textbooks on different pathological causes. Mental health is discussed by McMillan (2005). The "animals are not harmed if they don't know what they're missing" argument was first described by Crespi (1942) and is discussed more regarding wild animals by Mason (2006). The idea that "death is not a welfare issue" is best defended by Webster (1994) and an alternative by Yeates (2009b). Morgan and Tromborg (2007) provide a review of stresses caused by captivity. Isolation stress is discussed more by Sharp *et al.* (2002) and the effects of stresses by Moberg (2000). Iatrogenic harms are discussed more by Yeates (2012a).

Clients

2

2.1 Owner Causes of Feelings

Veterinary professionals are not the only humans with whom animals interact. Owners also affect their animals' feelings. What effect they have can depend on the legal status of the animals (discussed in Section 2.2), human–animal relationship (Section 2.3), and owners decision-making (Sections 2.4, 2.5 and 2.6), relationship with their veterinary professional (Section 2.7) and finances (Section 2.8). Depending on these factors, owners and carers can cause (or prevent) animals to experience many feelings that are worth avoiding.

Pain may be caused by injury or husbandry practices, and fear can be caused by negative or unpredictable stimuli, including painful interactions such as routine farm mutilations or inappropriate training methods. Pathological states can be caused by owners, for example by breeding that results in harmful diseases, and recent studies have suggested that these problems have been reported for many of the commonest pedigree breeds (Asher *et al.* 2009; Summers *et al.* 2010).

Hunger can be due to neglect or due to deliberate practices such as using broiler strains that make it necessary to starve breeding stock, breeding dairy cows whose milk-yields constitute excessive metabolic demands and forced moult methods in layers to increase productive lifespan. Similarly, overfeeding can be due to well-intentioned negligence, as with many companion animals, or deliberate, as in foie gras production. Discomfort can be due to lack of bedding, thermal extremes outside animals' thermal comfort zones (e.g. by failing to have

Animal Welfare in Veterinary Practice, First Edition. James Yeates.
© 2013 Universities Federation for Animal Welfare. Published 2013 by Blackwell Publishing Ltd.

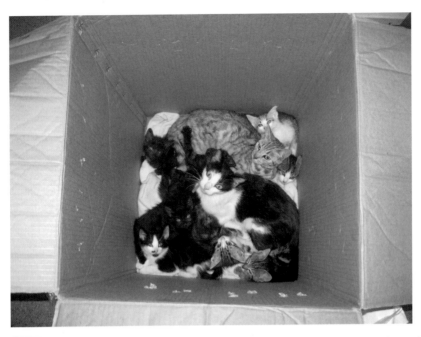

Figure 2.1 Owners may harm their animals by abandoning them, although relinquishing animals to charity centres may be better when owners cannot ensure their needs are met. (Courtesy of RSPCA Bristol.)

ventilation backup) or insufficient space, as is relatively common for rabbits in farm, laboratory and pet environments.

Suffering due to frustration may be caused by owners preventing animals performing motivated behaviours. Animals can be highly motivated to perform many *normal* or *natural* behaviours, and also many learned ones, and have general psychological needs such as choice, control and exercise. Conspecific interaction (with members of their own species) is important for members of gregarious species, such as sheep, pigs, chickens, cows, dogs, rabbits and horses, although many are kept in visual or tactile isolation. Human interaction is important for some individuals, such as dogs (Tuber *et al.* 1999; Odendaal 2000; Hennessy *et al.* 2002; Kobelt *et al.* 2003; Hiby *et al.* 2004; Coppola *et al.* 2006; Lefebvre *et al.* 2007), although many dogs are frequently left alone for long periods (PDSA 2011).

Owners sometimes also euthanase their animals prematurely, abandon them or relinquish them to shelters (Figure 2.1). Rescue shelters are a valuable way to give companion animals (and less commonly wild and farm animals) a second chance and to decrease abandonment. However, financial limitations can mean that animals' lives are compromised to varying degrees, despite the carer's best intentions (Tuber *et al.* 1999; Hennessy *et al.* 1997). In extreme cases, welfare problems can mean some animals would be better off euthanased than not provided with

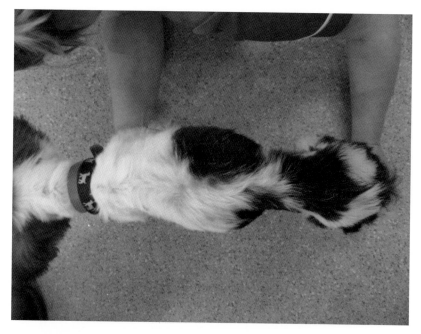

Figure 2.2 Owners may harm their animals by failing to provide enough resources. (Courtesy of RSPCA Bristol.)

adequate veterinary care, kept in overcrowded kennels with insufficient enrichment or kept beyond the time at which they should be euthanased (especially for wild animals who could not survive in the wild or farm animals that live beyond their natural lifespans). In less extreme cases, welfare compromises can decrease carers' ability to rehabilitate and train animals while also making it good for animals to be rehomed as quickly as possible.

Owners cause problems through their behaviours. Sometimes these behaviours are deliberate actions. Sometimes they are accidental. Sometimes owners neglectfully fail to act, and thereby to provide things that avoid welfare problems, while also preventing other people or the animal itself from doing so, such as when they underfeed an animal (Figure 2.2). As well as under-provision, owners cause harms by excessive provision (Figure 2.3), such as when they overfeed an animal (Figure 2.4). These distinctions are important in identifying *win-win* situations where improving animal welfare also benefits owners. Clients can also cause problems to animals they do not own (Figure 2.5).

Owner causes do not all involve pathological processes. Nevertheless, they are *contagious*. How people treat animals can spread to other people, through communicable attitudes, direct contact with established practices, purchases or laws (Table 2.1). In this way, welfare problems may spread like epidemics or become endemic in an industry (e.g. beak-trimming in the poultry industry) or within a

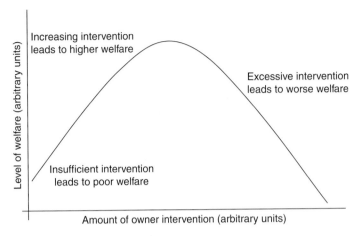

Figure 2.3 Representation of a theoretical relationship between level of owner interventions (e.g. provisions) and effect on animal welfare.

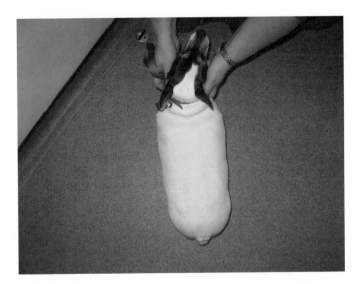

Figure 2.4 Owners may harm their animal by providing excessive resources. (Courtesy of RSPCA Bristol.)

small number of people (e.g. tail-docking amongst pedigree dog breeders), which then contaminates others (e.g. puppy buyers).

Fortunately, owners can also prevent and solve welfare problems and can be a useful source of enthusiasm, resources and solutions. Owners can also act to achieve good welfare for their animals, for example by providing them with exercise, mental stimulation and company. The behaviours that cause good welfare

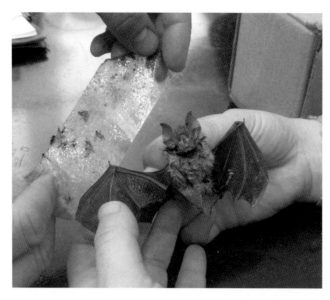

Figure 2.5   Clients can also harm animals they do not own, such as this bat caught in flypaper. (Courtesy of RSPCA Bristol.)

Table 2.1   Modes of transmission of contagious welfare practices.

Source	Mechanism	Example
Communicable attitudes	Communication of beliefs	Discussion fora (direct, social, internet)
Direct contact with established practices	Conscious imitation	Emulating good farms
	Accidental mimicry	Copying other jockeys' riding styles
Purchases	Positive reinforcement	Perpetuating intensive farming systems
Law-making	Negative reinforcement	Prohibiting onychectomies in cats

are also contagious and people can learn good practices from one another and from veterinary professionals.

Owners are responsible for how they treat their animals, whether well or badly. However, this does not mean that the veterinary professional does not have a responsibility *as well*. A veterinary professional has a responsibility to the animal, even if this involves *working on* as well as *working with* the owner. Unfortunately, each veterinary professional's animal welfare account is partly based on the animal welfare accounts of their clients.

2.2 Owners and the Law

How much veterinary professionals can achieve, and therefore for how much we can be responsible, depends on the circumstances. We are especially constrained by the law in each country, especially those relating to the legal relationships between owners and their animals and between veterinary professionals and their clients.

The legal relationships between owners and their animals in most countries usually give owners certain rights over their animals. The most obvious right is that of property. This allows owners to do many things to their animals, including sell them, use them, destroy them and to gain any benefits that derive from them.

In most countries, owners' property rights are not absolute. Sometimes owners can legally own animals only under certain conditions (e.g. licences for keeping dangerous wild animals). Often, owners cannot use their animals in any way whatsoever (e.g. owners cannot use their dog to kill their neighbour). Some laws can allow the state to deprive owners of their animal or to disqualify them from owning or using animals in the future, after their conviction for an offence.

In many countries, owners' rights are constrained by laws that protect the animals themselves. Owners are restricted by the generic laws described in Section 1.2, which apply both to an owner and anybody else's. Paradoxically, these laws may allow owners to harm their animals more than they can harm other people's, for example it may be legal for a farmer to put their own sow in a gestation crate but illegal cruelty for them to do it to someone else's. Some countries place more demanding legal responsibilities on owners to care for their own animals. In EU countries, farmers should take reasonable steps to protect the welfare of animals under their care and avoid those animals being caused any unnecessary pain, suffering or injury (Council Directive 98/58/EC). In the UK, such a duty of care applies to owners of all animals, who must ensure the needs of their animals are met to the extent required by good practice (Animal Welfare Act 2006).

Property laws also usually prohibit other people from doing things to someone else's animal. A person may be prosecuted in a criminal court if they take, destroy or damage another person's animal without their consent. A person may be sued in a civil court for any loss or damage. In most states, the compensation is usually relatively inexpensive, since most animals have limited financial value, but can often include any veterinary fees spent in repairing the damage.

Again, there are limits to the property right that prevents other people from damaging one's animals. For example, an owner's animal may be legally killed if it is considered dangerous (e.g. some dog breeds) or for disease control (e.g. in contiguous culling regimes). So veterinary professionals may be allowed to legally damage or destroy another person's property when they are acting on behalf of the government or when there is an overriding animal welfare concern, such as a suffering animal in an emergency situation.

Table 2.2 Elements of negligence in some countries.

Element	Meaning	Example of where may not apply
Duty of care	Veterinary professional must have some responsibility to the animal	Overriding legal duty, e.g. animal welfare
Breach of duty	Unreasonable failure	Mistakes
Harm done	A human, e.g. the *owner*, is caused harm that can be monetarily compensated	Where animal is harmed, but owner is not, e.g. lack of pain relief; veterinary surgeon provides free second surgery to repair iatrogenic damage

NB: This does not constitute legal advice, and the author cannot be held accountable for any decisions made. Readers are advised to consult a lawyer familiar with the jurisdiction in which they work.

Veterinary professionals may also destroy or damage another person's animal when they have the owner's valid consent. For example, if an owner gives you permission to kill their animal, they cannot later demand compensation, unless their consent is deemed invalid. Consent is usually valid if the person giving it is the legal owner of the animal (or their representative), sufficiently informed (e.g. about the operation), competent to give consent (i.e. can understand the information and make a decision) and free from undue influence (i.e. coercion). Consent allows an owner to refuse or permit treatment; it does not allow them to insist on it. So consent means a veterinary professional *can* do something; but it does not mean they *must*.

The ideas of property and informed consent underlie other legal duties that veterinary professionals have towards clients. Criminal laws may describe offences, such as theft and fraud or mandate actions such as data protection. Professional codes may add further duties such as honesty and confidentiality.

Owners also enter into legal relationships with veterinary professionals. These may be written contracts (e.g. in some horse vetting or some farm health planning schemes) but are often tacit or implied duty of care. Entering such relationships can place additional responsibilities onto the veterinary professional. As a specific example, owners can effectively delegate some of their animal welfare duties to veterinary professionals, so that the veterinary professional becomes responsible for their animals' welfare while they are in the practice, for example by providing food, shelter and, if necessary, emergency euthanasia.

Veterinary professionals' duty of care means that owners can bring claims against veterinary professionals for failing in that duty of care, for example through breaching confidentiality or negligence (Table 2.2). In many countries, veterinary professionals cannot be automatically successfully sued for every mistake (i.e. mistakes can happen without implying negligence), for any malpractice that does not cause the owner harm (i.e. there is nothing for which to compensate them) or for cases where their duties to the client are overridden by a greater responsibility. Crucially, this may allow situations where duty to their patient overrides duty to their client. This can allow veterinary professionals legally not to offer only options that lead to unreasonable welfare harms or to breach confidentiality to prevent future suffering by reporting an abusive client.

2.3 Owner–Animal Relationships

Owners' legal ownership of their animals forms a backdrop of their relationships with those animals, but there is more to owner–animal relations than simply that of property, and owners and animals can have very varied relationships (Figure 2.6). Human–animal relationships affect owners' husbandry methods, willingness to pay for treatment and likelihood to comply with advice. Understanding the different types of relationships can therefore be beneficial (Ormerod 2008) and help to achieve animal welfare improvements.

There are several useful ways to categorise human–animal relations. Often these are phrased in terms of how the humans regard the animals, e.g. as *companion animals* versus *farm animals* versus *laboratory animals* versus *wild animals*. These descriptions do not accurately map onto species (e.g. feral cats).

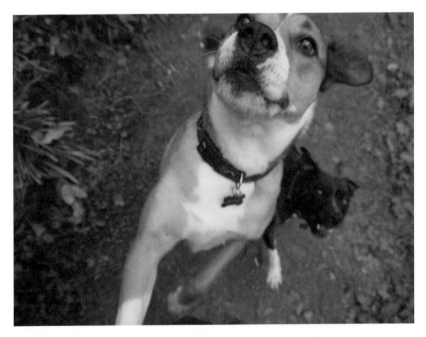

Figure 2.6 Animals have varying relationships with their owners. (Courtesy of James Yeates.)

Less commonly, animal–human relationships can be described in terms of how the animal regards humans, such as *tame* and *wild*.

Some owners relate to their animals personally, as individuals. This is well recorded for companion animals, especially in modern crazes like the furry babies movement and rites such as funerals and bar mitzvahs (Dresser 2000; Greenebaum 2004; Kenney 2004). Farmers may not think about farm animals in the same way, perhaps especially with regard to intensively farmed animals, since farmers may own millions of animals (Marcus 2005; Bock & van Huik 2007), and farmers are often described as thinking primarily in economic terms (e.g. Norton & Scheifer 1980; Wallace & Moss 2002). In fact, the situation is often more complex. Some companion animal owners think of their animals impersonally (e.g. puppy farmers) and some farmers relate to individual animals (Holloway 2001), such as in hand-rearing economically unviable orphan lambs (indeed, the term *pet* possibly originated from the term for such lambs).

One can think of human–animal relationships in terms of the animal welfare account owners have regarding their animal or in terms of whether each party is benefitted or harmed (e.g. by using terms from the ecological literature such as exploitative and symbiotic). We tend to think of companion animals as benefitting from humans and farm animals as being harmed, but owners' relationships with companion animals and farm animals may both be exploitative or symbiotic relationships, depending on the owner's welfare account towards the particular animal. One can also think of relationships in terms of dependency. Animals or humans are often *dependent* on each other for something they need (e.g. for food, survival or emotional support). Dependency does not necessarily imply that animals benefit – animals may be harmed by being dependent on humans if the humans do not provide what the animal needs.

One can also think of owner–animal relationship in terms of owners' moral viewpoints. Some may think that animals have a right to life or that they are completely disposable. Some may think they have equivalent moral status to humans, others that it is wrong to spend resources on them that could be better used on humans. Some may think that owners should have absolute property rights, others may think of their animals as colleagues. And owners can have very different attitudes to animal welfare and decision-making (Hemsworth & Coleman 1998; Boivin *et al.* 2003; Austin *et al.* 2005; Hemsworth 2007). These moral positions can obviously be different to our own, and sometimes in surprising ways, for example owners often consider killing an animal to be *cruel*, even where many veterinary professionals would consider keeping the animal alive to be cruel.

Characterising owner–animal relationships is useful but difficult. Different owners may have different relationships with different animals. Indeed, a single owner may have different relationships with the *same* animal. For example, an eventer may be a pet, a resource and a financial investment, and the owner may interchange or combine these relationships. Veterinary professionals need to recognise and respond to these different relationships.

2.4 Owner Decision-Making

Figure 2.7 shows a model of owners' decision-making. Understanding their decision-making process is vital for achieving good animal welfare, at all steps of their decision-making (Table 2.3).

The final step (Step 5) is the most important for welfare because it is an owner's behaviour that alters their animal's welfare. This behaviour may be straightforward, such as giving consent and payment, or it can be more demanding, such as committing to provide long-term aftercare. In some cases, this step can be emotionally charged, such as the act of killing an animal. Behavioural *changes* from previous behaviours may require some more demanding decision-making and particular motivation to maintain them.

Performing a desired behaviour requires that owners formulate a genuine intention to perform that action. In most cases, the intention occurs only just before the action. But sometimes, these two steps can be temporally separated. For example,

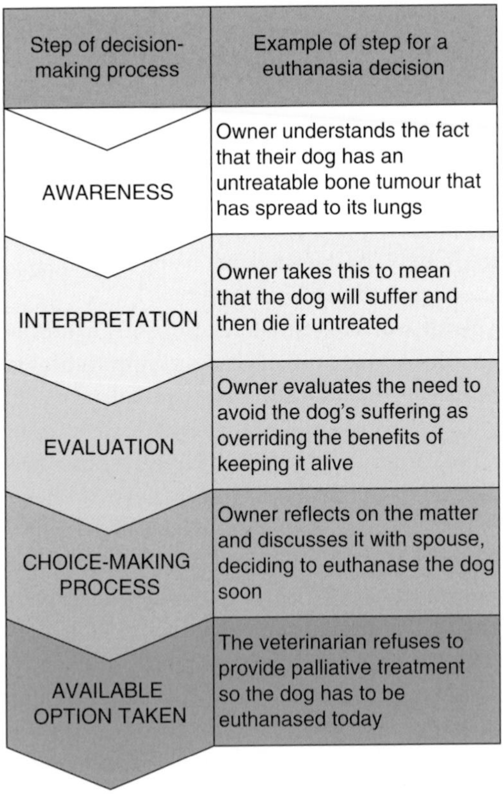

Step of decision-making process	Example of step for a euthanasia decision
AWARENESS	Owner understands the fact that their dog has an untreatable bone tumour that has spread to its lungs
INTERPRETATION	Owner takes this to mean that the dog will suffer and then die if untreated
EVALUATION	Owner evaluates the need to avoid the dog's suffering as overriding the benefits of keeping it alive
CHOICE-MAKING PROCESS	Owner reflects on the matter and discusses it with spouse, deciding to euthanase the dog soon
AVAILABLE OPTION TAKEN	The veterinarian refuses to provide palliative treatment so the dog has to be euthanased today

Figure 2.7 Model of owner's decision-making process. (Adapted from Yeates and Main 2011.)

Table 2.3 Useful information about owners.

Step of decision-making	Useful information
Awareness	Awareness whether there is a problem
Interpretation	Concerns about the animal
	Perception of the problem
	Ability to understand complex issues, uncertainties and risks, etc.
	Understanding of issues such as prognosis and cost
	Expectations of treatment regimes
Evaluation	Relationship
	Ethical values and principles
	Beliefs about animal welfare in general
	Other concerns, e.g. financial
	Motivations – benefits and barriers
Choice-making	Level of autonomy
	Desire to make decisions
Taking the chosen option	Resistance to change
	Ability to achieve outcomes

an intention to euthanase an animal may be made at home, but fulfilling that intention can involve both a time delay and a number of intervening steps. This gap allows owners to change their mind if the intention was not strong enough and the underlying reasoning was not sufficiently robust.

Forming an intention involves choosing from the range of options that are available (Step 4). Sometimes, owners' choices are based on their unreflective motivational emotional gut reactions, for example if they have a phobia about one option (e.g. due to previous experiences) or when their emotions do not allow them to consider an option (e.g. to lose a beloved pet). Our motivational set-up has been created through millennia of evolution and years of experience, so it should be relatively reliable and efficient, but its quickness may make it inaccurate. But they can depend on many psychological and other factors, including owners' risk-aversiveness (Potter & Gasson 1988; Brotherton 1989; Willock et al. 1999a,b; Austin et al. 2001; Vanslembrouck et al. 2002; Edwards-Jones 2006).

Owners' choices may also depend on social norms, based on what (they think) other people think they should do (Fishbein & Ajzen 1975). Owners are influenced by people close to them, including friends, family and partners (couples often appear to be trying to second-guess each other's view, especially if they have not discussed a decision until the consultation). Owners are particularly influenced by their peers such as other farmers or riders. Dog owners compare themselves to other dog walkers. Farmers often look around each others' farms. Owners' choices are also influenced by experts such as veterinary professionals, who can be described as *key opinion leaders* because our messages and opinions are especially

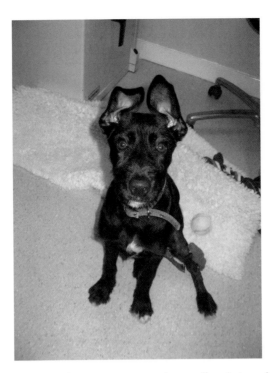

Figure 2.8 Owners' emotional responses to animals can affect their evaluations. (Courtesy of RSPCA Bristol.)

authoritative. Owners are also influenced by society at large, via laws and widespread social morals. These motivations can lead to conflicts when people try to please multiple people who have differing views.

Before making a choice, owners may evaluate the benefits and barriers of each option (Step 3), in order to formulate an attitude towards each option (Ajzen & Fishbein 1980). This evaluation relies on owners' emotions. These may be *current emotions*, such as love and pity (Figure 2.8), *retrospective emotions*, such as regret, or *prospective emotions*, such as fear or hope. These emotions are coloured by the owner's background *moods* such as happiness, depression and anxiety, which may make an owner more optimistic, pessimistic, risk-prone or risk-averse. In turn, these moods are affected by owners' previous emotions. Used unreflectively, owners' emotions are like text messages. They are quick and personally relevant to the owner and their animal, which makes them useful ways to make fast decisions. But emotions can be unsophisticated, personal and often seem like complete nonsense to others, which makes discussions about evaluations difficult where unempathetic people share different attitudes or where one party talks only about the facts and ignores the contested emotional elements.

In some cases, owners may make decisions by considering what affective emotions they would expect to experience for each option. Specifically, people may evaluate decisions in terms of the likelihood of them later *regretting* their decision (Larrick & Boles 1995; Ritov 1996). The motivation not to speed may come not from the risk of killing someone but from the risk of regretting having killed someone (see Parker *et al.* 1996). A similar evaluation may underlie some owners' decisions against euthanasia, where people are concerned about regretting their decision at a later date, and this seems intuitively more likely for an irreversible decision, such as euthanasia. In one sense, this involves empathising with one's future self. Similarly, owners may make evaluations based on what is expected to avoid guilt. Guilt relates to social norms, although guilt is an effective motivator only if the person genuinely considers an action to be wrong. For example, in one study many people showed no evidence of guilt from extending the life of terminally suffering animals (Brockman *et al.* 2008). Thus, persuading such owners is unlikely to succeed by merely pointing out the suffering or the social norm.

Owners' evaluations can also depend on their personality. For example, a person's self-esteem can affect how risk-averse they are. People with lower self-esteem may be more averse to risky actions (when they expect feedback on the outcomes). Conversely, people with higher self-esteem may be more risk-seeking (Josephs *et al.* 1992). Interestingly, people may also take more risks if they are less socially accountable (Tetlock & Boettger 1994).

Owners make evaluations based on their interpretation of the evidence (Step 2). Owners' interpretations may be based on unreflective empathy, their *lay knowledge*' about health and welfare and their anthropomorphic reasoning. Lay knowledge can be incorrect and uninformed, but a lot of research in the human field has considered patients' decisions to add a valuable dimension to clinical decision-making (e.g. Stacey 1994; Williams & Popay 2006).

Before owners can interpret evidence, they need to be aware of it (Step 1). This first step is vital. If owners do not even perceive a problem, then it is unlikely that they will even begin to follow the steps towards making a decision. This can make it important, if unexciting, for veterinary professionals to encourage owners to observe their animals, learn about preventative health methods and look for changes and problems. However, owners may resist awareness of an issue and seem to deliberately fail to recognise a problem. For example, owners may resist acknowledging a problem because they fear that doing so will lead to a decision to undergo risky or expensive treatment. Owners' later steps can affect their earlier steps because they learn from their previous decisions and can predict their later decision-making.

2.5 Owner Benefits to Improving Welfare

It is useful for veterinary professionals to identify ways in which improving animals' welfare also benefits their owners. As Chapter 5 will describe, this information can be used to achieve welfare goals. Three important types of benefits are those that improve the owner's own health, finances or general well-being.

There is an increasing amount of work on the benefits of animals to human health, and this is now a specialism within psychotherapy (although see Herzog 2011). Much of this work unfortunately pays insufficient attention to the welfare of the animals that can be quite badly harmed (Brody 2011). In many cases, improving an animal's welfare can also increase an owner's health. For example, owner obesity appears to be linked to canine obesity but not feline obesity, suggesting that increasing exercise for dogs may also improve an owner's health (Nijland *et al.* 2010). Similarly, better training or socialisation may decrease anxiety and reduce fear-related aggression or the risk of a rider falling off. Helping owners to improve animal welfare can therefore improve owners' health.

Often improving welfare can lead to financial benefits. Some welfare improvements can lead to later economic savings, for example through prophylactic interventions such as vaccination, ovariohysterectomy, good nutrition or breeding strategies. Other welfare improvements can improve animals' fertility, productivity or performance, for example herd health planning and husbandry changes to decrease lameness or mastitis can both reduce pain and increase milk-yield. Welfare investments can also make animals more sellable when consumers pay more for healthier animals, for example through repairing or preventing congenital problems and appropriate socialisation. Helping owners to improve animal welfare can therefore improve those owners' wealth.

Improving welfare can also provide owners with a *feel good* factor. Improving animal welfare allows empathetic owners to enjoy seeing their animals happy and contented and avoid seeing them suffer. Improving animal welfare allows owners to enjoy social approval and praise and avoid feeling guilt, regret, embarrassment or shame. In extreme cases, improving animal welfare allows owners to avoid prosecutions, which can lead to owners losing their animals, receiving criminal records, paying fines or serving prison sentences. Helping owners to improve animal welfare can therefore make those owners feel good too.

Improving welfare can also improve owner–animal relationships. For example, animal behavioural problems affect the owner and the animal. Some may cause self-harm. Some may signify unpleasant feelings such as fear or distress, either at the time or previously, or underlying pathologies. Aggression in animals may be due to medical problems, such as cranial nerve deficits, hepatic encephalopathies, inflammatory processes and of course pain, especially aural, dental, gastrointestinal or pancreatic pain. Separation-related behaviours may be due to anxiety and include many behaviours that are indicative of stress (Appleby and Pluijmakers 2003), including vomiting/diarrhoea (Takeuchi *et al.* 2001) and repetitive behaviours (Borchelt and Voith 1982; Luescher *et al.* 1991, 2005) (c.f. McCrave 1991). Solving behavioural problems may improve welfare if it ameliorates the underlying feelings and helps owners to enjoy their relationship with their animals.

2.6 Owner Barriers and Biases

Owners often face various barriers to improving their animals' welfare, at all stages in the decision-making process.

At Step 1, owners are unaware that there is a welfare problem in the first place (even some issues that seem blatantly overt to experienced assessors). Owners often miss welfare issues that occur during their absence (e.g. separation-related behaviours or horses running out of food overnight) or before the animal is even purchased (e.g. poor breeding practices or lack of juvenile socialisation). Owners may be especially likely not to notice subtle symptoms or gradual changes, e.g. degenerative disease or obesity (Figure 2.9), or to spot when a normal behaviour *stops*. Unawareness can be due to ignorance (e.g. not knowing what is normal), emotional biases (e.g. not wanting to see a problem that could prompt euthanasia) or underlying attitudes (e.g. lack of caring). From an animal welfare perspective, it is not important whether the ignorance is excusable but whether it is remediable or preventable.

At Step 2, owners might notice that there is an issue but misinterpret its welfare implications. Misinterpretation can be due to a lack of background information, for example when owners are unaware of the possibility of prophylactic treatment. It may also be due to erroneous information. Clients have increasingly more sources

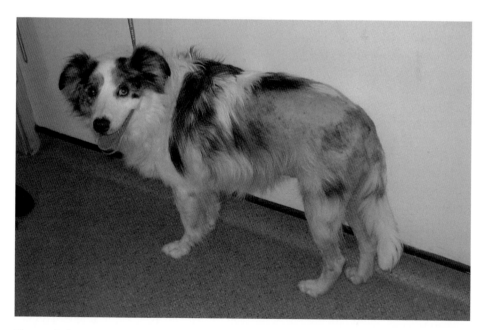

Figure 2.9 Owners may fail to notice (or to act on) gradually worsening problems. (Courtesy of RSPCA Bristol.)

of information (Blackwell 2001) and higher expectations (Antelyes 1990), and these may not be accurate or realistic. Misinterpretation can also be due to excessive emotion, for example when owners are too emotionally overwhelmed to engage, or due to insufficient emotion, such as lack of empathy (especially in males; Heleski *et al.* 2005) or failure to emotionally engage, in a similar way to how non-vegetarians can emotionally *detach* themselves so that they can eat meat without being concerned or feeling guilty.

At Step 3, owners can make an erroneous welfare evaluation. Some people have less concern than others for animals (Kellert & Berry 1987; Herzog *et al.* 1991; Furnham & Heyes 1993; Hills 1993). Some owners focus on only certain aspects of welfare, such as physical health or certain feelings such as pain, or consider death to be more harmful than suffering, which effectively rules out euthanasia. Owners may also excessively focus on short-term harms or benefits and rate far-future events and far-past events as less important. In particular, recent feelings have more effect on people's assessments (Suh *et al.* 1996; Heinonen *et al.* 2004), and this may bias treatment decisions, such as euthanasia (McMillan 2007). Humans also struggle to understand probabilities (Hastie & Dawes 1988). Another common error is to continue treatment in order to justify having already provided treatments despite the fact that these are *sunk costs*, in terms of either previous expenditures or previous animal welfare harms.

One general phenomenon reported for owners' evaluations of future welfare is the *disability paradox*. Healthy human patients tend to rate the effect of a pathology or disability as more significant than patients with that condition. For example, people imagine spinal injuries would be devastating, but people with spinal cord injuries actually report similar levels of quality-of-life to healthier people (Whiteneck *et al.* 1992; DeLisa 2002; Hammell 2004). An equivalent finding has been reported for owners' perceptions of paraplegic dogs' welfare (Bauer *et al.* 1992), and owners can have similarly exaggerated concerns over dogs' blindness (Chester & Clark 1988; McMillan 2007) or limb amputation (Withrow & Hirsch 1979; Carberry & Harvey 1997). A similar finding is called a *response shift*, in which people alter their assessments as time goes on, usually resetting their assessment criteria to compensate for changes, so that they have a new baseline for what is an acceptable or good quality-of-life.

At Step 4, some owners fail to make a welfare-friendly choice because they place their own interests above those of the animal. Some owners want to make or save money, to keep their animals in their own possession or to avoid demanding effort or lifestyle changes. For example, Heleski *et al.* (2005) found economic concerns to be the most common type of barrier to farm animal welfare improvements. It can be a barrier for one owner to be at home to administer twice daily treatments or to walk their dog daily. What an owner chooses can depend on what *competitor behaviours* they would do instead of the welfare-friendly behaviour. What an owner chooses can also depend on their perception of the animal (e.g. some owners opt for euthanasia because they see their animal as a disposable economic unit or as theirs alone) and themselves (e.g. other owners pay for expensive treatment because they see themselves as self-sacrificial and payment reaffirms their self-sacrifice). Some owners may be unable to make a choice at all, for example consenting to euthanasia, even if they have evaluated it as the best option for the animal.

At Step 5, owners might make a decision but be unable to achieve it, for example in cases of poor compliance with treatments. This may be due to simply forgetting and due to later reconsidering their earlier decision because they did not really endorse the decision itself at a deep enough level.

Thus, there is a temptation to consider that finances are the main barrier to veterinary treatment, but barriers can occur at all stages. This fits with findings in other areas. For example, it appears that the main barrier against consumers buying animal-friendly products is not normally the cost of the higher welfare food but the lack of information about the welfare-friendliness of the production method to help consumers decide how to spend their money (Eurobarometer 2007). This is a useful lesson for veterinary professionals.

2.7 Vet–Client Relationships

Owners' decision-making forms a backdrop of our relationships with them. Clinician–client relationships affect how much veterinary professionals can achieve animal welfare goals and how much clients are willing to pay for treatment and comply with advice. Understanding the different types of relationships can therefore help to achieve animal welfare improvements.

There are several useful ways to categorise client-clinician relations. Often clients are classed in terms of their animals or human–animal relationships, e.g. pet owners versus breeders versus farmers. We can also relate to people as *owners* versus *clients*, each of which have different implications for their legal status and their role in animal welfare improvements.

We can think of client–clinician relationships in terms of who benefits and loses. Veterinary professionals can benefit financially, through job satisfaction, feeling good or satisfying our intellectual curiosity. Clients can benefit when we keep their beloved animals alive; increase animals' commercial value or productivity; save clients money; avoid them feeling guilt, worry or grief, etc. We can also define client–clinician relationships in terms of how we balance benefitting clients with benefitting patients. We can be collaborators for the client's wishes, promoting their interests even when these conflict with the patient's welfare. We can be advocates for the animal's interests, promoting their welfare even when these conflict with clients' interests.

We can also think of clients in terms of *how* they are relevant to improving welfare. We can think of owners as *part of the problem*, who need to be advised and manipulated, or as *part of the solution*, who can be worked with openly and constructively. One approach is to think of ourselves as helping clients to fulfil

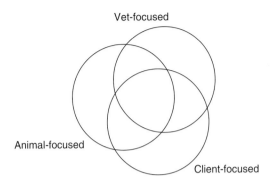

Figure 2.10 Good decision-making can help to make the clinician's, client's and animal's focuses coincide.

their animal welfare responsibilities as owners. When clients are concerned with their animal's welfare, advocacy and collaboration are in parallel and vet-focused, client-focused and animal-focused motivations are in parallel (Figure 2.10). In other cases, achieving animal welfare goals may involve going against clients' wishes, but we can still consider such efforts as benefitting clients insofar as they help people to do their duty as owners.

Client–clinician relationships can vary in terms of the clinician's moral views towards clients' wishes. Owners can place veterinary professionals under considerable pressure, for example towards prescribing antibiotics, authorising a controlled muti-lation, conducting performance-enhancing surgery, keeping quiet about a criminality, offering free treatment, falsely signing a certificate perpetuating the life of a suffering animal or terminating the life of a healthy one (Yeates & Main 2011b). Sometimes paternalistic veterinary practitioners may think that clients should unthinkingly fol-low their instructions regarding their animals. Veterinary professionals are authorita-tive and trustworthy persons and what they say can command considerable respect. In other cases, veterinary professionals may think that autonomous clients should be unthinkingly respected regarding their property. Clients are competent, rational and intelligent people and what they say should determine what happens. In between, clients and veterinary professionals can both contribute to a joint concordance. In fact, there is a continuum of different clinician–client relationships (Box 2.1).

Owners are not simply people who implement our decisions (or not). They are individuals who make their own decisions, and it is those decisions that determine what they do. Crucially, owners need to formulate a behavioural intention to act in the necessary way (Ajzen 2005). This intention is more than a belief that they should do it or even desire to do it (and certainly more than having received an instruction to do it). Getting owners to form the right intention requires treating them as individuals. This means that there is no right clinician–client relationship. Different approaches may be better in different situations and different decisions and with different owners.

Box 2.1   Models for clinician–client relationships.

Technician	*Veterinary professional unquestioningly fulfils owner's wishes*
Facilitator	*Veterinary professional assists owner to make their own decision, by giving them necessary information but leaving the decisions to the owner*
Partner	*On model that best decisions are where veterinary professional and owner combine in joint decision-making*
Advisor	*Veterinary professional guides owner to make their own decisions, by giving them the necessary information and influencing their decision-making*
Arbiter	*Veterinary professional gets information from the owner, but makes own decisions and tries to achieve those decisions through persuasion, etc.*
Enforcer	*Veterinary professional knows what is the best course of action without consultation and tries to achieve those decisions through persuasion, etc.*

2.8 Money Problems

As one specific example, many veterinary conflicts concern money. On one side of the transaction, owners want medical treatment but have to pay when they buy veterinary services. Sometimes owners expect treatments to provide financial returns by making their animals more valuable (e.g. cosmetic or performance-enhancing surgery) or avoid future costs (e.g. vaccination to prevent disease). At other times, owners buy treatment out of concern for their animal's welfare. On the other side, practices want to improve their patients' welfare but have to charge when they sell veterinary services. Veterinary practices are also motivated to promote welfare, but they must cover costs, get a fair wage for their expertise, fund practice investment and ideally generate profit. Veterinary professionals might be tempted to provide treatment to increase profit, especially if they are partners or on profit-related-pay.

The two sides of the transaction can create conflicts between the client versus the veterinary practice, between the owner versus their animal or between the veterinary professional versus their patient. This conflict can mean that welfare is not always maximised, for example treatments may be provided to make the clients or the practice money, or avoided in order to save money. Efficiency drives may lead to mistreatment, for example reduced consultation times may prevent effective investigation, leading to misdiagnoses or effective client communication, leading to lower compliance.

Competition between practices can also prevent veterinary professionals from achieving their welfare goals. Practices need to retain clients and to remain competitive with other practices, and it can be difficult to maintain one's welfare-focus and remain competitive. For example, one may think an option is against a patient's interests, but refusing to provide it would be ineffective if other colleagues or nearby practices will provide the treatment. So veterinary professionals may perform a given intervention (e.g. euthanasia), because they think that otherwise a colleague will do so. This could lead to a *race to the bottom*, in which many veterinary practitioners provide treatments they consider imperfect, because they think others will otherwise do so.

In an ideal economic model, vet–client transactions should constitute a compromise that optimises both sides' interests. But the veterinary industry has many market imperfections. Clients are not ideal informed consumers and rely on veterinary advice to make decisions, so transactions are not equal exchanges. Clients cannot easily shop around since veterinary prices are hard to compare without understanding what therapies involve and differing standards of care. In some cases, veterinary practices make it even harder by discounting conspicuous items as loss leaders (e.g. neutering) while retaining higher prices for other services (e.g. emergency treatments). Moreover, some owners may be prepared to pay virtually unlimited fees, not always due to insurance, which removes a barrier to excessive treatment.

Even if veterinary markets functioned perfectly, they would balance the interests of the client and the practice, but they would not maximise animal welfare. Economic theory suggests that financial transactions will maximise the benefits to the humans directly involved in the transaction and not the animal – animal welfare is an *externality* or side effect that affects non-transacting parties. In addition, veterinary fees correspond to the cost of a therapy to the veterinary professional (e.g. in time or training), rather than its value to the animal (in welfare improvements). To put it another way, fees pay for veterinary services, not for animal health.

These problems can have animal welfare implications. As an obvious example, some owners will not be able to fund necessary treatment. In these situations, practices can, and do, provide pro bono work. However, as commercial companies, practices cannot afford to provide widespread pro bono services (and doing so might encourage irresponsible ownership) and doing so could reduce a practice's efficiency and thus competitiveness. Other owners can fund treatment. While pet ownership can span many different socioeconomic groups (Westgarth *et al.* 2007; Murray *et al.* 2010), many pet owners have few animals and relatively high incomes (Goodwin 1975; Endenberg *et al.* 1992), and many owners report they would spend any amount on their companion animal (Albert & Bulcroft 1987). This helps their animals, but the fact that different animals with the same condition can receive different amounts of treatment may seem unfair (Yeates 2011a).

Summary and key recommendations

- Owners and carers can cause, prevent and solve problems through their behaviours and have an animal welfare account towards their animals. Owner behaviours are *contagious*. Achieving animal welfare improvements has to involve working with owners. Clients can be part of the problem and part of the solution.
- Civil duties and property law can limit our options but often do not prevent welfare-focused practice. Veterinary professionals can treat people as clients and as owners. Consent allows an owner to prevent treatment but not to insist on it. Both the owner *and* the veterinary professional have responsibilities to our patients.
- Clients make their own decisions. Owners' decisions can be modelled as awareness, interpretation, evaluation, choosing and achieving. Owners can benefit from improving animal welfare (e.g. health, wealth and happiness) but they face barriers to doing so (e.g. finances and time). Owners also have barriers and biases in their decision-making, including non-welfare-focuses.
- Veterinary practice can be client-focused, vet-focused or welfare-focused.

Selected further reading

There are tens of animal welfare books on different owner causes. Good starting points are Fraser and Broom (2008), Webster (2005) and Yeates (2012a) and the journals *Animal Welfare* and *Applied Animal Welfare Science*. On more specific issues, German (2006) looks at obesity, McGreevy *et al.* (2011) at riding and Rooney *et al.* (2007) at training.

Human–animal relationships are discussed by several authors (Dollin 1999). Farmer attitudes are reviewed by Edwards-Jones (2006). The importance of property status is discussed by Radford (2001), with alternative views given by Francione (1994), Tannenbaum (1995) and Tischler (1977). The benefits of animals to human health are described by Herzog (2011) and Fine (2010) and on the SCAS website (http://www.scas.org.uk/1851/benefits-of-the-bond.html). Owners' relationships with their animals as individuals are recoded for companion animals by Brockman *et al.* (2008), Irvine (2003, 2007) and Taylor (2007). The *furry babies* movement is described by Greenebaum (2004) and mourning for animals by Dresser (2000) and Kenney (2004). Holloway (2001) describes how some farmers do relate to individual animals, but the opposite is suggested by Bock and van Huik (2007) and Marcus (2005). The role of veterinary professionals in improving this relationship is described in AAHABV (1998), Rollin (2006a) and Lue *et al.* (2008).

Human decisions and behaviour are discussed generally by Ajzen (2005). More specifically, the role of emotions in reasoning is discussed by Damasio (1995) and

LeDoux (1998) and predicted regret in particular by Larrick and Boles (1995) and Ritov (1996). The role of empathy and lay knowledge about health are well described in Blaxter (1983), Davison *et al.* (1991) and Illman (2004) with demonstrations of lay knowledge's validity provided by Stacey (1994) and Williams and Popay (2006). Ainslie (2001) discusses the issue of reasoning about future events. Brockman *et al.* (2008) consider owner decision-making. The disability paradox is discussed by LePledge and Hunt (1997) and Ubel *et al.* (2005) and applied to animals by McMillan (2007), and a generally enjoyable exploration is provided by Gilbert (2006).

Welfare Assessment

3

3.1 Patient Assessment

The last two chapters have said a lot about animal welfare problems, and the next three will say more about how to achieve welfare improvements. But how can we identify problems or improvements? Both require some method of assessing welfare. In the first case, we need some way to *screen for* potential problems or opportunities. In the second case, we need to *gauge* welfare, in order to say whether an animal's welfare has been (or will be) made better or worse. This chapter focuses on how we can make these assessments.

Welfare assessments can help practitioners to keep sight of their aim to improve welfare, focus on both medical and non-medical issues and avoid being overly distracted by trying to satisfy clients. Welfare assessment may provide useful information, such as prognostic indicators to predict disease progression (Rumsfeld *et al.* 1999; Kaplan *et al.* 2007). It can also improve owner engagement and clinician–client relations, as described in Chapter 5.

The steps involved in welfare assessment can be modelled as in Figure 3.1, which match the steps described earlier for owners in Figure 2.7. Step 1 involves gathering information through history-taking, clinical examination and further tests (discussed in Sections 3.2, 3.3 and 3.4). Step 2 involves interpreting that information into presumed feelings, using inductive and deductive methods (Sections 3.5 and 3.6). Step 3 is to evaluate those presumed feelings into an overall welfare assessment, using qualitative or quantitative methods (Sections 3.7,

Step of decision-making process	Methods	Example of step for a euthanasia decision
INFORMATION GATHERING	History–taking Clinical examination Further tests	One identifies that a dog has radiographic signs of a bone tumour and is limping
INTERPRETATION	Empathy Induction Hypothetico-deduction	One interprets this to mean that the dog is experiencing pain
EVALUATION	Qualitative methods Quantitative methods	One evaluates that the suffering is overriding the benefits to the dog of remaining alive

Figure 3.1 Model of animal welfare assessment by veterinary professionals.

and 3.8). Sometimes these steps can be combined into more formal assessment methods (Section 3.9).

Screening for problems involves only Steps 1 and 2 of welfare assessment. Screening does not involve an overall evaluation but highlights issues for further investigation. It is useful during routine consultations such as vaccinations or geriatric health-checks, and it can encourage owners to consider issues such as diet, parasite control, osteoarthritis and exercise. Screening can also be used to monitor for disease alterations and treatment side effects.

In comparison, gauging welfare involves all three steps of assessment. Gauging welfare does involve an evaluation, so it assesses which treatment options will provide the best welfare for the patient. It can encourage owners to make decisions and provide consent. Gauging can also be used to monitor disease progressions, improvements or deteriorations and treatment effects.

The different steps in assessment provide scope for possible errors and disagreements between different people. Evidence of such differences in veterinary contexts is relatively unstudied, but one veterinary research paper incidentally reported some differences between proxies in assessing demeanour (Graham *et al.* 2002) and similar disagreements appear common in human medicine. Many veterinary professionals can recall examples where their assessments have disagreed with those of owners, paraprofessionals or colleagues. Disagreement may occur during any step of the assessment process.

In Step 1, people may have different information. For example, an owner may have seen what the animal is like at home but not in surgery. They may be unaware of diagnostic facts or have failed to notice a behaviour or symptom. Differences in memory can mean that people forget information, or that they forget what an animal's welfare was like previously, especially if there has been a gradual decline or improvement. People may also have incorrect information through unfounded assumptions or misinformation.

In Step 2, people may interpret the available information differently, due to different levels of empathy or abilities to understand scientific knowledge. They may have different ideas about what information is important, e.g. whether pathophysiological or behavioural indicators are more important. They may have different background knowledge or experience. They may also have different knowledge of the individual patient.

In Step 3, people may use different methods of evaluation. People have varying opinions on how worthwhile feelings are (e.g. whether pain is more important than fear). They may be biased by personal interest; for example, a desire to justify continued treatment may predispose them to rating welfare as disproportionately high. People may impose their own values (e.g. needle-phobia), have different personal experiences or undergo a response shift.

Welfare scientists have spent a lot of time designing and validating assessment methods to reduce these disagreements. Inter-observer and intra-observer reliability are suggested as key attributes of a good welfare assessment method. Such consistency is useful to make farm assurance schemes more fair, to evaluate welfare variations when assessors change (e.g. between nursing shifts) and in experiments and clinical trials that need to be repeatable. Reliability is actually less important in veterinary practice: what is important is accuracy (and if an assessment is *wrong*, reliability simply means that it is consistently wrong).

The possibilities of disagreements and errors raise the question of *who* is best placed to assess welfare. Veterinary surgeons will generally have more experience of welfare assessment than owners. Veterinary nurses and owners may spend more time with an individual animal and have more knowledge of the animal's inputs, behaviours and individual personality. Different assessors may therefore be better placed in different cases. More importantly, collaboration can combine all the valuable information, interpretations and evaluations from every contributor.

Veterinary professionals can contribute a lot to such joint assessments. For Step 1, we can provide clinical knowledge and diagnostic skills. For Step 2, veterinary professionals have experience of interpreting information about diseases and clinical symptoms into animal's feelings and using scientific methods and critical anthropomorphism. For Step 3, veterinary professionals can help to guide the partnership through an appropriate evaluation process. In all steps, veterinary professionals can also help to correct errors that owners may make and provide encouragement and support. The rest of this chapter goes through the steps of welfare assessment, suggesting ways in which veterinary professionals can make accurate and reliable welfare assessments.

INFORMATION

3.2 Histories

Box 3.1   Four (+one) questions concerning what information is worth obtaining for clinical decisions.

(1) What is important for the animal?
(2) What information is available to us?
(3) What available information will help us to make decisions?
(4) What iatrogenic harms might assessment methods cause?
(5) (For gauging welfare) Is the information measurable over time?

The first step in animal welfare assessment is to work out what information to obtain. There is no point in trying to get information that is irrelevant, unavailable or meaningless – in busy veterinary practice, we only just have enough time to assess the things that are worth assessing. Determining what to assess involves four (or five) questions, listed in Box 3.1.

Question (1) has been answered in Chapter 1. What is important to an animal is the valence and intensity, duration and frequency of its feelings, and the achievement or avoidance of anything that causes or signifies such feelings. Question (2) means we must focus not on trying to directly *see* animals' feelings, but on available information about *inputs* and *indicators*. We cannot see a cow's pain, but we can detect a sole ulcer, which may cause it, or non-weight-bearing, which may indicate it. Question (3) reminds us to focus on information that helps us make practical decisions for the animal's benefit. We may require different information depending on whether we want to screen for problems or to gauge welfare, on how we plan to interpret and evaluate the information and on what decision we have to make. Question (4) reminds us that diagnostics may be harmful if they require repeated visits, restraint or anaesthesia, and these risks need to be balanced against the benefits of the information (Question (5) will be discussed in later sections).

Before the consultation, clinical records can provide information about an animal's or herd's previous problems, geographical location, vaccination history, previous vet-fear or in-practice aggression, signalment (e.g. its age, gender, and breed) and the owner's other animals. Further valuable information is usually provided by the owner's opening statement, which can reveal the owner's animal welfare assessment, priorities and personal motivation. Owners may not present all welfare issues, especially problems they do not feel are *veterinary* issues, such as fear-related or separation-related issues.

Veterinary professionals therefore need to actively gather more information about the animal's inputs (Box 3.2) and indicators (Box 3.3), especially the animal's

Box 3.2 Inputs relevant to history-taking.

- Disease
  - Congenital
  - Acquired
  - Old age
- Disability
- Injury
- Abuse
- Inter-animal aggression
- Nutrition
  - Poisons
  - Insufficient water
  - Insufficient food
  - Inappropriate food
  - Excessive food
  - Enjoyable food
  - Unpleasant food (e.g. eating unpalatable medicines or while nauseous)
  - Force-feeding
- Environment
  - Risks of injury
  - Insufficient bedding or thermal extremes
  - Lack of space
  - Being unable to predict their environment
  - Interruption of normal routine
  - Threatening stimuli
  - Novelty
  - Inability to control their environment
  - Kennelling
- Conspecific company
  - Positive interactions
  - Isolation
  - Aggression
  - Loss of resources
- Human company
  - Rewards/enjoyable interaction
  - Company of usual carer
  - Abuse
  - Punishment
  - Humans associated with previous negative or positive interactions
- Company of other animals
  - Predation
  - Loss of resources

- Treatment
  - Transport
  - Visiting the practice
  - Restraint
  - Punishment
  - Hospitalisation
  - Anaesthesia
  - Surgery
  - Medications

Box 3.3   Responses relevant to history-taking (may be increased or decreased).

- Vomiting, diarrhoea and imbalance
- Grooming, licking and scratching
- Repetitive behaviours
- Eating and drinking
- Weight changes
- Sleeping
- Activity and willingness to exercise/go out
- Engagement with toys and play
- Interaction with other animals, including allogrooming
- Responses to humans, including willingness to interact and specific responses to human approach
- Altered posture
- Paw-lifting and pawing
- Frequency and types of vocalisations
- Escape behaviours
- Shaking or trembling
- Hiding
- Gait, soundness and ease of movement
- Guarding a particular area, and prayer-posture
- Grooming, licking and scratching at a particular area
- Overall demeanour
- Any other abnormal behaviours
- Any other unnatural behaviours
- Any other behaviours

current levels and recent changes. These should be related to the *individual* patient's preferences, fears and likes. Relevant information includes facts about the owner, such as their beliefs about animal welfare and how they assess it, their level of care and knowledge, their planned inputs and what recommendations they are likely to

> **Box 3.4 Five freedoms** (after FAWC 1992).
>
> - *Freedom from thirst, hunger and malnutrition* – by ready access to fresh water and a diet to maintain full health and vigour
> - *Freedom from discomfort* – by providing an appropriate environment including shelter and a comfortable resting area
> - *Freedom from pain, injury and disease* – by prevention or rapid diagnosis and treatment
> - *Freedom to express normal behaviour* – by providing sufficient space, proper facilities and company of the animal's own kind
> - *Freedom from fear and distress* – by ensuring conditions and treatment which avoid mental suffering

> **Box 3.5 Five opportunities** (after Parker and Yeates 2012).
>
> - *Opportunity for selection of dietary inputs* – by provision of a diet that is preferentially selected
> - *Opportunity for control of environment* – by allowing the achievement of motivations
> - *Opportunity for pleasure, development and vitality* – by maintaining and improving beneficial inputs
> - *Opportunity to express normal behaviour* – by providing sufficient space, a proper range of facilities and the company of the animal's own kind
> - *Opportunity for interest and confidence* – by providing conditions and treatment which lead to mental enjoyment

comply with and what they want and expect. Some information can be obtained by explicit, if tactful, questions. Other information needs to be indirectly inferred, by mindreading through similar critical reasoning to how we infer animals' feelings.

There are many potential barriers to obtaining information through owners. Owners may fail to provide information about certain issues through not observing, recognising or remembering them. Owners may also misreport issues through poor memory, misinterpretation or dishonesty. Some owners may deliberately hide information, for example if they think revealing it could lead to legal prosecution, moral criticism or a euthanasia decision. Other barriers are due to *our* limitations. We may interrupt, misinterpret and fail to ask, listen, follow-up or remember. We may lack enough time to collect sufficient information, especially when owners are particularly recalcitrant or loquacious. We may make erroneous prejudgements or assumptions about situations and owners.

Veterinary professionals can gain more information efficiently by using pre-organised frameworks. One can structure discussions around frameworks such as the five welfare needs (Box 1.2) or focus on feelings and causes, such as the five freedoms (Box 3.4), perhaps supplemented with five opportunities to consider positive welfare as well (Box 3.5). Different questioning techniques can be useful in different cases (Table 3.1). Alternatively, owners can be asked to complete a

Table 3.1 Methods of questioning.

Method	Closed or open	Definition	Examples	Where useful
Binary questions	Closed	"Yes"/"No" questions	"Is your cat vomiting?" "Do you vaccinate against condition X?"	Screening for specific issues (e.g. known side effects or contraindications)
Quantitative questions	Closed	Questions that ask for an objective measurement	"How many litres of water does your horse drink each day?" "How long has that chicken been lame?"	Assessing against set parameters (e.g. species normal values or previous measures)
Relative questions	Closed	Questions that ask for an evaluation relative to something else	"Is your cow milking normally, less or more?"	Assessing change over time where previous value unknown
Qualitative questions	Open	Questions that allow the owner to choose from (effectively) unlimited options	"How has your rat been acting recently?" "How would you consider your dog's quality-of-life?"	General screening Rapid gauging
Undefined questions	Open	Questions that allow the owner to interpret the question	"How is your rabbit?" "How are your lambs doing?"	Opening statements Screening

paper-based questionnaire before the consultation. An example for dogs is given in Figure 3.2 that looks at specific responses and welfare needs.

3.3 Clinical Examinations

One can also gain information from examination (Figure 3.3). It is useful to first look at the animal's overall demeanour, and then at more general symptoms of arousal and valance.

Closer clinical examination can provide evidence of causes of welfare problems. Disease can be assessed by feeling or listening for abnormalities (e.g. a mass or an irregular heart-beat). Injuries can be inspected visually or palpated. Nutrition can be assessed using bodyweight and body condition score. Hydration can be assessed by checking mucous membranes (Pritchard *et al.* 2005) and skin turgor. Examination can also provide an idea of whether the condition is acute or chronic.

Please remember to mark these lines according to how much of a problem they are *for your dog*, not for you. Please place a mark (X) where on the line that represents how much of a problem each of the following issues are for your dog at the moment. Then, for each one please tick whether you think the problem has changed from last time you were asked. Please tick whether it has (1) worsened, (2) not changed or (3) improved.

Fear – of noises, people or in stressful situations – trembling, dribbling, tail tucked under or attempts to escape

No problem   **Major problem**

From last time you were asked, do you think your dog's fear level has   *1. Worsened* ☐   *2. Not changed* ☐   *3. Improved* ☐

Anxiety – *over-dependency or clinging; noisy, destructive or unsettled, e.g. when left alone*

No problem   **Major problem**

From last time you were asked, do you think your dog's anxiety level has   *1. Worsened* ☐   *2. Not changed* ☐   *3. Improved* ☐

Senility – *disorientation, decreased alertness or responsiveness, altered sleep patterns, loss of housetraining*

No problem   **Major problem**

From last time you were asked, do you think your dog's senility has   *1. Worsened* ☐   *2. Not changed* ☐   *3. Improved* ☐

Itchiness – *including nibbling, scratching, head shaking*

No problem   **Major problem**

From last time you were asked, do you think your dog's itchiness has   *1. Worsened* ☐   *2. Not changed* ☐   *3. Improved* ☐

Breathing problems – *including coughing, sneezing, trouble breathing*

No problem   **Major problem**

From last time you were asked, do you think your dog's breathing has   *1. Worsened* ☐   *2. Not changed* ☐   *3. Improved* ☐

Figure 3.2 Assessing owners' perceptions of dog responses and needs. (Adapted from Mullan and Main 2007.)

Eating, drinking and vomiting problems – *including excessive drinking or eating and loss of appetite*

No problem   Major problem

From last time you were asked,
do you think your dog's eating, etc. has   *1. Worsened* ☐   *2. Not changed* ☐   *3. Improved* ☐

Toileting problems – *including diarrhoea, pain, incontinence*

No problem   Major problem

From last time you were asked,
do you think your dog's toileting has   *1. Worsened* ☐   *2. Not changed* ☐   *3. Improved* ☐

Mobility problems – *including unwillingness to exercise, stiffness, problems getting up*

No problem   Major problem

From last time you were asked,
do you think your dog's mobility has   *1. Worsened* ☐   *2. Not changed* ☐   *3. Improved* ☐

Unsociability – *including aggression; lack of independence*

No problem   Major problem

From last time you were asked,
do you think your dog's unsociability has   *1. Worsened* ☐   *2. Not changed* ☐   *3. Improved* ☐

Weight – *including overweight and underweight*

No problem   Major problem

From last time you were asked,
do you think your dog's weight has   *1. Worsened* ☐   *2. Not changed* ☐   *3. Improved* ☐

Other problems *(e.g. other medical and behavioural conditions)*

No problem   Major problem

From last time you were asked,
do you think this problem has   *1. Worsened* ☐   *2. Not changed* ☐   *3. Improved* ☐

Figure 3.2   *(cont'd)*

Dog Welfare Needs Assessment

In this section, please describe your dog's usual situation.

1. Environment (*where your dog spends most of its time*)

Where does your dog sleep at night?	....
Where does your dog stay during the day?	....

2. Exercise and activities (*your dog's walks and work – where, when, how often, for how long and amount of freedom on walks*)

What exercise does your dog get?	....
For how long?	....
How often?	....
What other activities does your dog enjoy regularly?	....

3. Diet (*what, when and where your dog eats and drinks, your dog's food and water*)

What is your dog's diet?	....
How much does your dog get daily?	....
How often?	....
What other food does your dog get?	....

4. Mental stimulation (*your dog's play, training, toys*)

What opportunities does your dog have for mental stimulation?	....
How often?	....

5. Companionship

What companionship with other people does your dog get?	....
How often?	....
For how long?	....
What companionship with other dogs does your dog get?	....
How often?	....
For how long?	....

Figure 3.2 (*cont'd*)

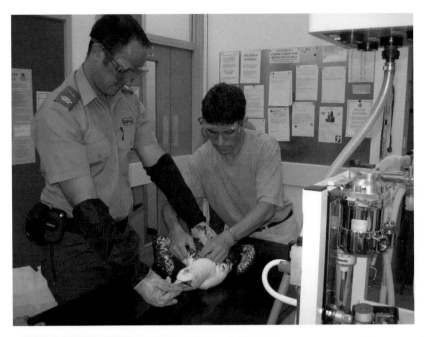

Figure 3.3 Veterinary professionals can obtain information on causes and symptoms from clinical examination. (Courtesy of RSPCA Bristol.)

Clinical examination includes observation of animals' physiological symptoms, both general and local. Clinicians can assess an animal's immune system (e.g. inflammation, lymph gland enlargement, discharges and pyrexia), endocrine system (e.g. heart rate and dermatology), renin-angiotensin system (e.g. hydration and skin turgor), cardiovascular system (e.g. heart rate and mucous membranes) and nervous system (e.g. lameness, guarding or licking at an area and vocalisations), as well as specific symptoms such as chromodacryorrhoea (the red tears that can be an indicator of stress in rats) and local symptoms such as erythema (redness) and swelling. Measures of sympathetic activation can indicate arousal, using inexpensive methods such as temperature, pupil dilation, heart rate and respiratory rate (plus each can be altered by pathological processes). As suggested in Chapter 1, many animals are iatrogenically aroused by being at the veterinary practice, so these measurements may simply indicate vet-fear and should be interpreted accordingly.

Clinical examination also includes observing behavioural symptoms, both spontaneous and induced. Clinicians can assess locomotive activity, limb withdrawal, vigilance behaviours and responses to objects or people. For example in horses, locomotive activity may be an indicator of stress (Houpt & Houpt 1989), responses to human approach or contact with areas such as head or chin may indicate fear (Pritchard *et al.* 2005) and pawing or snorting may indicate stress (Visser *et al.* 2008).

Clinicians can use formalised methods to quantify particular issues. Emaciation can be assessed using bodyweight, girth or standardised body condition scores. Pain is one phenomenon for which no simple, objective measure has been identified (Rutherford 2002), but one can nonetheless assign scores (Hawkins 2002). There are also frameworks for assessing pruritus, disease severity, fractures and many clinical issues, as well as overall welfare, quality-of-life or health-related-quality-of-life scoring systems (see further reading). Clinical examination often compares findings to what is normal for the individual, breed or species, usually based on the practitioner's experience.

One advantage of using clinical measures is that they seem to be more objective and more scientific than qualitative judgements. However, there can still be differences between assessors. For example, Burn *et al.* (2009) reported that assessments of body condition were sufficiently reliable for clinical use, but that assessment of hoof quality, hock injuries, mucous membrane abnormalities and skin tenting were not. One disadvantage of using clinical findings is that they may lead to an excessive focus on pathophysiological issues. This may be especially likely for veterinary professionals, who have scientific and medical backgrounds (McMillan & Rollin 2001). This problem is also recorded in the medical profession (Bradley 2001), where doctors can thereby miss opportunities to achieve other welfare improvements.

Another disadvantage of clinical examinations is that they require handling and restraint, which can cause stress, especially when the test is particularly strange (e.g. tonometry to measure intraocular pressure), when the animal is in an unusual environment (e.g. a darkened consulting room), or when the veterinary staff are stressed themselves (e.g. by time constraints or an uncooperative patient). Some tests are unpleasant in certain situations, such as testing an animal's pupillary light reflex (how their pupils react to changes in light intensity) if the animal is photophobic, or pain withdrawal assessment. In some cases, remote examination from a distance or from outside the cage can gain information before or instead of physical restraint. In other cases, sedation or anaesthesia may be less harmful than conscious handling. In some cases, it may be better not to perform a full examination or to delay some handling until after administering analgesia or anaesthesia.

3.4 Further Investigations

Clinicians can also obtain information from further tests such as laboratory tests, imaging, electrographics (e.g. electrocardiograms to assess heart function) and specialist physical examination tests. Further tests usually look for deviations from physiological normality. In some cases, there are lists of normal parameters for various populations. In other cases, one can use comparisons to the individual's normal state, for example by referring to previous radiographs of the same area or contralateral radiographs of the animal's healthy side.

Table 3.2 Example uses of further tests as welfare measures in and outside veterinary practice.

	Veterinary animal welfare assessment: pathological states	Veterinary animal welfare assessment: non-pathological states	Animal welfare science assessment
Imaging	Pathologies Organ size	*To be developed*	fMRI Adrenal size

Biochemistry	Endocrine or organ
	  function tests
	Specific immune
	  responses
		Hyperglycaemia	HAC assays
			  adrenaline

Haematology	Infection Blood disorders	*To be developed*	Stress leucogram Leucocyte carrying capacity
Electrography	Heart function Deafness	*To be developed*	EEGs
Post-mortem	Gross changes	*To be developed*	Gross changes
Behavioural **tests**	Sensory function tests	Eating Local pain responses	Preference tests Fear tests

As Table 3.2 suggests, there are lots of measures that veterinary surgeons use to identify specific welfare harms due to pathologies and lots of animal welfare measures that are used in fields outside veterinary practice. Contrastingly, there are few non-pathological measures used in veterinary practice for welfare assessment.

Biochemical and haematological measures can be assessed by analysing animals' blood samples and can provide information about the welfare of animals as diverse as horses (Hamlin *et al.* 2002; Robson *et al.* 2003) and ball pythons (Kreger & Mench 1993). Veterinary professionals often measure biochemical and haematological values as routine screening or as tests for conditions such as inflammation, dehydration and acidosis (where the animal's blood pH is too acidic).

Veterinary practitioners usually assess hypothalamo-adreno-cortical (HAC) axis responses to evaluate endocrine functioning. Animal welfare scientists use the same hormonal measures to assess non-specific stress responses in both the short term (e.g. increased cortisol, corticosterone and their metabolites) and long term (e.g. altered ACTH-stimulation or dexamethasone-suppression tests), measured in the saliva, plasma, serum, urine or faeces. Plasma cortisol assays can be done through most practices' commercial laboratories, but are relatively expensive, especially considering that most animals in a practice or during an intervention are likely to be stressed, making an elevated cortisol level of limited usefulness.

In comparison, clinicians (and animal welfare scientists) do assess moderate hyperglycaemia (high blood sugar) and glycosuria (sugar in the urine) as a measure of stress in cats. However, we often fail to consider the welfare implications; indeed,

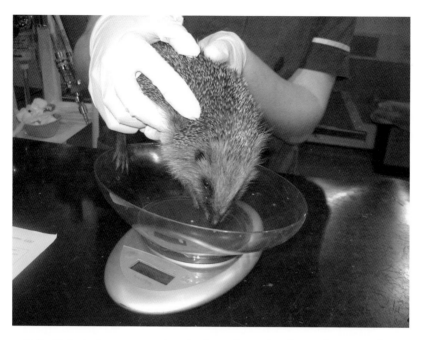

Figure 3.4 Biological measures such as bodyweight can be objectively measured over time. (Courtesy of RSPCA Bristol.)

we often deliberately *ignore* stress-induced hyperglycaemia, because we are focusing on assessing endocrine function and describe it as spurious. But such hyperglycaemia actually provides a useful indication that a cat is stressed, which should confirm the importance of considering the manner and frequency of rechecks and further tests (and the lack of hyperglycaemia may make us feel more tests may be less iatrogenically harmful). It may be true that feline hyperglycaemia is common in veterinary practices, but this highlights how many cats routinely experience vet-fear.

Further behavioural tests are also underutilised in veterinary practice. These are often done unthinkingly, such as offering an animal food to assess appetite or water-intake to assess polydypsia (increased drinking). Practitioners could similarly identify individual animal's preferences by providing a choice, for example by offering a hospitalised cat a variety of types of food or bedding. Observing animals' behaviour during hospitalisation can provide us with valuable information about its stress, apathy, vet-fear, frustration and sociability, so that we can adopt our husbandry accordingly.

One advantage of biological measures is that they often use standardised clinical or quantitative laboratory techniques. This can limit controversy about whether an animal is in a particular state and can objectively monitor changes over time (Figure 3.4). One disadvantage is that such parameters are not directly important to the patient, so practitioners still need to consider how they indicate feelings, and this may be more controversial.

INTERPRETATION

3.5 Empathy and Knowledge

The next step is to interpret information about inputs and indicators into what feelings they may cause or signify. This is not always simple. Like other clinical tests, welfare parameters can vary in their sensitivity (how often they recognise a problem) and specificity (how often they recognise the absence of a problem). Some symptoms may have a number of differential diagnoses, and some may not directly represent any feelings at all, for example if they signify benign pathologies. Plus, welfare assessments often involve combining various bits of information and its interpretations, which are often not easily comparable, and different sources of information may lead to conflicting evaluations (Mason & Mendl 1993; Fraser 1995).

Veterinary professionals can interpret information using only their direct empathy. Some studies have suggested that qualitative empathetic interpretations are more reliable than one might expect and often correlate with more objective welfare measures (Wemelsfelder *et al.* 2001; Wemelsfelder 2007). Veterinary professionals may have different levels of empathy (Herzog *et al.* 1989), and some may be relatively unempathetic (O'Farrell 1990), perhaps due to the effect of veterinary education (Paul & Podberscek 2000). Consequently, empathy alone does not provide a definitive assessment (Figure 3.5).

Fortunately, interpretation can be improved by the use of background knowledge. Published scientific data can improve interpretation, although there is a relative lack of scientific data about non-health-related aspects of animal welfare within veterinary practice. Because scientific methods cannot directly observe feelings, background scientific information is most useful to relate inputs and indicators such as symptoms, diagnoses, aetiologies, risk factors, possible treatments and sequelae that are later caused by the pathology. It is clinicians' own judgements that determine how to apply scientific evidence to particular cases.

Another source of background information is one's experience of one's own feelings and evidence of those of other humans, extrapolated through critical comparative reasoning in egomorphism and anthropomorphism. This makes it useful to consider how humans are caused feelings (Table 3.3) and how they respond (Table 3.4). Human–animal comparisons also allow us to adapt approaches that assess human quality-of-life for use in veterinary practice, so long as we adequately reflect human–animal differences. A large amount of work has gone into developing tools to assess human quality-of-life, although there is still no universally agreed framework for assessing human quality-of-life (Bowling 2005).

Just as the ultimate comparison begins with an individual (oneself), it also ends with an individual – the particular animal. Welfare interpretations should recognise differences between individuals. Animals, like humans, vary in their likes, fears, preferences, knowledge, biology and underlying conditions. For example, if an animal has hyperadrenocorticism (Cushing's syndrome) or cerebellar hypoplasia,

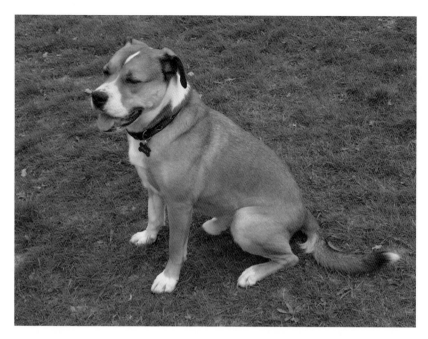

Figure 3.5 Direct empathy does not always provide a definitive welfare assessment. (Courtesy of James Yeates.)

Table 3.3 Example inputs that may be inferred, based on critical anthropomorphism, to cause feelings in animals.

Cause	Effect of presence	Possible effect of absence
Disease and injury	Pain, malaise, pruritus, etc.	Feeling of vitality?
Presence of (perceived) danger	Fear	At ease, unperturbed
Nutrition and hydration	Satiety, over-fullness	Hunger, thirst
Novelty	Interest, excitement, fear	Relaxation, boredom
Predictability of environment	Anticipation, feeling of control	Anxiety
Control of environment	Feeling of control	Feeling of lack of control
Fulfilment of motivation	Satisfaction	Frustration
Previous rewarding events	Optimism	Pessimism
Previous aversive events	Pessimism	Optimism
Repeated/previous success	Confidence	Lack of confidence
Presence of offspring/mother	Affection, love	Anxiety, lack of soothing
Conspecific company	Affection, friendship, fear of aggression	Loneliness
Interspecific company	Affection, friendship, fear of aggression	Loneliness
Exercise	Entertainment, fatigue	Restlessness
Warmth	Thermal comfort, overly hot	Feeling cold
Sex (when wanted)	Euphoria, love	Sexual frustration (not pre-adolescent)
Space	Feeling of freedom	Feeling trapped

Table 3.4 Example symptoms that may signify feelings in animals.

Symptom	Possible underlying feelings	
	If symptom is increased relative to normal	**If symptom is decreased relative to normal**
Overall demeanour	Various	Various
Escape behaviours	Aversion, pain, fear (*flight response*)	Aversion, pain, fear (*freeze-response*), apathy
Lethargy or increased sleeping	Malaise, pain, fatigue	Hypervigilance/stress
Locomotion – towards something	Excitement, interest, motivation Fear (aggressiveness)	Aversion, fear, apathy
Locomotion – away from something	Fear, play	Confidence, apathy, play
General activity	Fear, play, excitement, disorientation, seizure	Apathy General anaesthesia, coma, death
Head-pressing or guarding	Pain	–
Self-administration of analgesics	Pain Addiction	Lack of pain, lack of awareness of benefit
Vocalisations	Various	Various
Vomiting , regurgitation or hypersalivation	Nausea Var. pathological conditions	(Ruminants or feeding birds) Hunger or var. pathologies
Heart rate	Excitement or fear Var. pathological conditions	Low arousal Var. pathological conditions
Plasma/urine/faecal/ salivary cortisol	Excitement or fear Var. pathological conditions	Low arousal Var. pathological conditions
HAC function (cortisol or altered regulation)	Sustained stress Cushings disease	Sustained stress Addison's disease
Engagement with toys	Enjoyment, curiosity, investigation or fear	Apathy, bored with those toys, fear of toys
Shaking or trembling	Coldness or high arousal, e.g. fear or excitement (neurological conditions or fever)	(Neurological conditions)
Scratching at area	Pain, pruritis, stress	Adequate analgesia
Licking lips	Gustatory pleasure or discomfort on lips	Discomfort on lips
Generalised licking	Pruritis (e.g. skin or hepatic disease), distress, dirtiness	Lethargy, malaise
Any activity in a given situation	Motivation to perform that activity in that situation	Apathy

then one might not interpret high cortisol as stress or trembling as coldness or fear. A clinician's interpretation of the welfare of one patient may therefore come to different conclusions than the same clinician's assessment of another animal.

3.6 Induction and Deduction

Interpreting causes and symptoms can be done informally and unreflectively, using one's natural empathy. However, interpretation may be more accurate if it is based on a more *scientific* method. Veterinary professionals might use two methods that parallel the inductive and hypothetico-deductive methods of science described in Chapter 1.

Using an inductive method involves several steps. A clinician firstly obtains all potentially relevant pieces of information through screening and then compares the findings to evidence of relationships between them. For example, if a dog is vocalising (e.g. barking, howling or whining), destroying things, urinating, defecating or vomiting indoors or showing repetitive behaviours within 30 minutes of having been left alone, then comparison with published evidence (e.g. Blackwell *et al.* 2003) suggests that this is separation-related behaviour.

Less commonly, inductive methods can be used to relate findings to published data or experience about animals' feelings. If evidence suggests that certain symptoms are associated with a situation that would be expected to cause a feeling, then those responses may be interpreted as signifying those feelings in other contexts (Figure 3.6). For example, rabbits are observed to freeze and then perform escape behaviours in a predator's presence, which may be expected to signify fear, and similar behaviours in a veterinary clinic may be interpreted as signifying fear. In other cases, we may have observed our own behaviours to be associated with certain emotions (e.g. shaking with fear), which we then egomorphically extrapolate to other animals.

Inductive methods have several advantages. Screening can help practitioners to consider a range of aspects of an animal's life. Where there are published studies available, inductive methods allow the practitioner to make some interpretations without using any empathy or critical anthropomorphism. They need only to evaluate the quality of the evidence and decide how the evidence fits the specific case. They can then use statistical and probability-based reasoning to decide what the information may mean. It therefore fits with evidence-based veterinary medicine.

However, inductive methods also have limitations. For many issues, the scientific evidence base is still far from completion. Even when it is possible, screening and evidence searches are costly in both time and money. Asking a whole series of questions can take longer than a 10 minute consultation allows. Performing multiple investigative tests is expensive. Long and complex screening tools may even disengage owners. Screening methods can be especially inefficient when they do not fit with owners' natural ways of interacting with veterinary professionals, or when they do not fit with the clinician's ways of thinking. In addition, inductive methods cannot take into account the individuality of animals' preferences and responses to treatment.

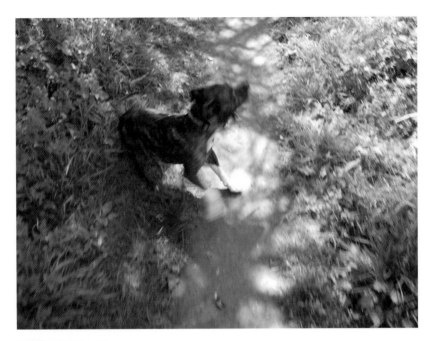

Figure 3.6 Symptoms must be taken in context. Repetitive spinning may indicate a neuropathy or stereotypy, but this dog is on a walk in which he otherwise appears very excited. (Courtesy of James Yeates.)

An alternative method of interpretation is to use hypothetico-deductive reasoning similar to the hypothetico-deductive method of designing scientific studies. This effectively involves conducting a mini experiment. A clinician first generates general hypotheses about what the animal's welfare might be like and then uses critical anthropomorphism, previous scientific reports and experience to identify what information would support or refute the general hypothesis. If such evidence is forthcoming, then this supports the hypothesis; if not, the hypothesis is thrown into question. As an example, a clinician might generally hypothesise that after being spayed, a cat may feel pain, and then look for pain-related behaviours such as licking the area, lethargy or hyperactivity, etc. If the cat does show such symptoms, this supports the hypothesis; if not, we should question the interpretation that it is in pain.

Hypothetico-deductive methods have several advantages. They can be efficient, focused and can show you are listening to the owner. The hypothetico-deduction process focuses down, using previous answers to generate new hypotheses, which are then tested by more detailed questions. It can start with an appreciation of the animal's overall demeanour, which is often described in terms of an underlying feeling, such as *excited*, *bored*, *listless*, *restless*, etc., and then to test increasingly specific hypotheses.

However, hypothetico-deductive methods involve several risks. If a practitioner does not think of a particular hypothesis, they will not test it and so will fail to make the correct interpretation. Another risk is that a practitioner may interpret

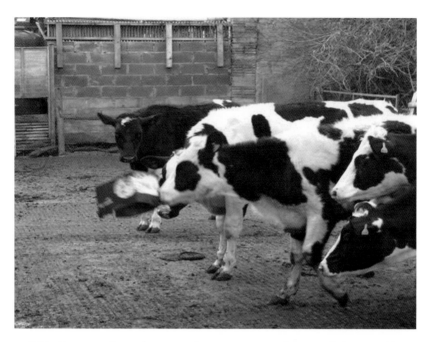

Figure 3.7 Playing with an object may be a symptom and cause of pleasure. (Courtesy of James Yeates.)

evidence in a biased way that tends to support their hypothesis – what the psychology literature calls *confirmation bias*. To avoid this, it is usually sensible to entertain multiple competing hypotheses concurrently and to perform some screening alongside deductive questions.

In practice, veterinary professionals should use a combination of inductive and deductive methods. For example, one can screen for issues and use this to identify hypotheses for more focused investigation. This can allow particular respondents to give detailed information without asking the same questions of every respondent and without potential information being excluded by presumptive diagnoses and biased interpretation.

For both inductive and hypothetico-deductive methods, it can be useful to group inputs and symptoms according to the hypothesised type of feeling that they support. This is commonly done for behaviours. *Pain-related* symptoms include inactivity, aggression, vocalisations, postural changes, self-trauma, response to analgesia, etc. (Sandford *et al.* 1986; Potthoff & Carithers 1989; Hellyer & Gaynor 1998; Firth & Haldane 1999; Taylor & Weary 2000; Holton *et al.* 2001; Taylor & Robertson 2004). Fear or anxiety-related symptoms include lowered posture, aggression, startling, vocalisations, vigilance, paw-lifting and body-shaking (Beerda *et al.* 1997, 1998, 1999). Malaise symptoms include lethargy, apathy, stress leucograms, dehydration and sickness behaviours (Hart 1988). Pleasure-related causes and symptoms include play (Figure 3.7), allogrooming and vocalisations

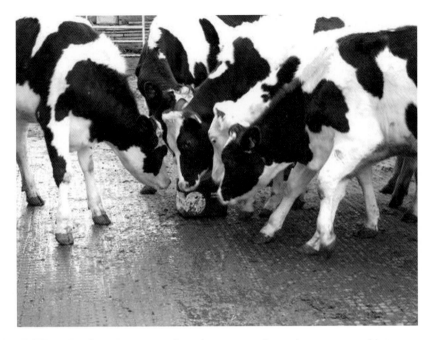

Figure 3.8 Animals' investigation of an object may indicate they are enjoyably interested in it. (Courtesy of James Yeates.)

(Boissy *et al*. 2007b; Yeates and Main 2008). Interest is indicated by approach and investigation (Figure 3.8). Table 3.5 suggests some feelings that might be inferred from inputs, based on critical anthropomorphism, the published scientific literature and the author's experience.

EVALUATION

3.7 Qualitative Welfare Evaluation

Once the information has been interpreted, it is necessary to evaluate the patient's welfare in terms of whether it is good or bad. One way to do this is to use qualitative assessment methods. Qualitative methods are commonly used by owners and by veterinary professionals as well.

The simplest qualitative measure is whether an animal's welfare is *good* or *bad*, using open questions such as "How do you feel your animal's quality-of-life is?" or "How is the herd's general welfare?" To assess change over time, one can ask whether the animal is better or worse, as in Figure 3.9. This comparison can be improved by minimising response shift by explicitly recalling certain events, by using photographs, or by using a list of objective binary symptoms (e.g. eating?), which they can easily identify when absent.

Table 3.5 Inputs and associated feelings.

Inputs	Example specifics	Likely feelings	Example indirect effects	Likely feelings
Disease	Congenital Acquired Old age	Pain, malaise, nausea, pruritus, frustration	Disability	(See disability)
			Altered physiological responses, e.g. polyphagia or polydypsia	Hunger, thirst
			Sequelae, e.g. gastric ulceration	(See disease)
Disability	Poor mobility	Frustration, confusion, boredom	Long-term recumbency or inactivity	Discomfort
			Bed sores	Pain
	Inability to urinate	Discomfort, pain	Inappropriate urination/ defaecation	Discomfort
			Poor communication	Fear (see injury)
Injury	Abuse Accidental injury	Pain, fear	Aggression to humans/other animals	(See injury)
Diet	Poisons or inappropriate food	Nausea, pain, confusion	Disease	(See disease)
	Insufficient water	Thirst	Dehydration	Thirst, malaise
	Insufficient food	Hunger, malaise, pain	Deficiencies, e.g. hypoglycaemia	Fatigue (see disease)
	Excessive food	Overfullness	Obesity	Breathlessness, fatigue (see disability)
			Diabetes	Thirst (see disease)
			Dystocia	Pain, fatigue
			Raised expectations	Frustration
	Unpleasant food	Unpleasant taste	Decreased intake	(See insufficient food)
			Not taking medicines	(See disease)
	Force-feeding	Nausea, discomfort	Increased intake	(See excessive food)
	Enjoyable food	Gustatory pleasure, satiety		

(continued)

Table 3.5 (cont'd)

Inputs	Example specifics	Likely feelings	Example indirect effects	Likely feelings
Environment	Insufficient bedding	Discomfort	Injury or disease	(See disease) (See injury)
	Thermal extremes			
	Lack of space	Frustration	Obesity	(See obesity)
	Unpredictable environment	Fear, anxiety	Risks of injury	(See injury)
	Interruption of normal routine		Conditioned learning against objects	Fear, apathy
	Threatening stimuli			
	Inability to control their environment			
	Novel or unusual events	Pleasure Fear	Conditioned learning towards objects	Pleasure
	Rewarding objects	Pleasure		
Company of other animals (conspecific or interspecific)	Friendly interactions (e.g. allogrooming/ allopreening)	Pleasure	Conditioned learning towards conspecifics	Pleasure
	Isolation	Frustration, loneliness	Lack of communication skills	(See aggression)
			Lack of habitation	Fear, anxiety, lack of confidence
	Aggression	(See injury)	Expectation of injury	
	Predation		Conditioned learning against conspecifics	
	Competition for resources	Frustration	Aggression	(See aggression)
			Lack of resources	(See diet) (See environment)
			Disease risks	(See disease)
Human company	Friendly interactions	Pleasure	Conditioned learning towards humans	Pleasure
	Abuse Punishment	(See injury)	Conditioned learning against humans	Fear, anxiety

(continued)

Table 3.5 (cont'd)

Inputs	Example specifics	Likely feelings	Example indirect effects	Likely feelings
Treatment	Transport	Nausea, fear	Conditioned learning	Fear, anxiety
	Visiting the practice	Fear	Conditioned learning	Vet-fear
	Restraint	Fear, frustration		
	Punishment	Pain, fear, frustration		
	Hospitalisation	Fear, frustration	Altered nutrition	(See diet)
			Altered environment	(See environment)
			Company of other animals	(See company of other animals)
			Company of humans	(See company of humans)
	Anaesthesia	Dysphoria		
	Surgery	(See injury)	Inflammation	(See injury)
	Medications	Nausea, unpleasant taste	Not taking medicine	(See disease)

These two questions are about assessing your dog's quality-of-life as a whole.

Please put a mark (X) to describe how your dog has been recently and circle whether you think this has (1) worsened, (2) not changed or (3) improved.

A. All things considered, how contented do you think your dog is?

Very content or happy   Very discontent or miserable

Since the last time you were asked,   1. Worsened ☐   2. Not changed   3. Improved ☐
do you think your dog's contentedness has   ☐

B. All things considered, how willing would you be to take on the life your pet is now living? (X)

Completely willing   Completely unwilling

Since the last time you were asked, are you   1. Less willing ☐   2. Equally   3. More willing ☐
                                                                       willing ☐

Figure 3.9 Questionnaire for assessing dog owners' overall qualitative evaluations. (Adapted from McMillan 2003 and Mullan and Main 2007.)

Qualitative evaluations lack transparency, which makes it hard to resolve disagreements or to make joint assessments. In some cases, it may therefore be useful to consider a more explicit or objective basis for overall evaluations. One example is hierarchical assessment methods. These put different inputs or states in an explicit order of importance, and evaluate each animal's welfare in terms of which level of the hierarchical scale it reaches. For example, if good health is considered to be a more important input than company, then an animal that has good health but no company is said to have better welfare than one with company but poor health. Hierarchical approaches would evaluate the welfare of a herd based on the level of its worst-off member.

Hierarchical frameworks suffer from two problems: one minor and one major. The minor problem is deciding what things are more important. It may be possible to place feelings in a hierarchy. Others have suggested lists of causes or feelings that are the most important, often described as needs. However, there is limited agreement about what really constitutes a need and the concept itself remains vague and relatively unhelpful without further explanation.

One useful distinction for veterinary professionals is between *vital needs* and *psychological needs*. Vital needs are whatever is necessary for life to continue, such as nutrition (or food), hydration (or water) and respiration (or oxygen). Psychological needs are whatever is necessary to avoid suffering, such as the absence of (too many) harmful inputs and the ability to perform highly motivated behaviours. Often, the same things are required to satisfy both vital and psychological needs, for example eating food is necessary both to live and to avoid hunger. In other cases, different things are required to satisfy vital and psychological needs, for example where avoiding suffering requires either death (e.g. euthanasia) or a risk of death (e.g. letting a cat out with a risk of road accidents). In these cases, opinions may differ as to which need is more important.

Alternatively, we may think we cannot place vital and psychological needs in a hierarchy. This highlights the major problem for hierarchical methods: it is not easy to defend ranking things into a consistent hierarchy at all. In general, we may judge some things as more important, for example many people think health is more important than aesthetic appearance. We may also base a hierarchy on biological observations that some motivations can occur only if more *pre-potent* ones are satisfied or if some other states are absent. For example, play may only occur when basic needs for food are satisfied (Hurnik & Lehman 1988) and if the animal is not in significant pain or fear (Fraser & Duncan 1998). Similarly, starved humans appear to lose interest in any higher aspirations (Keys *et al.* 1950).

However, such generalisations are too simplistic. Priorities vary between animals, between contexts and over time. Food may be more important than water for an animal that is well hydrated but starving, but water is more important for an animal that is well-fed and dehydrated. People voluntarily undergo anaesthesia and cosmetic surgery, and grooming may be very important in some cases (Figures 3.10 and 3.11). It is also not apparent that there are motivations that

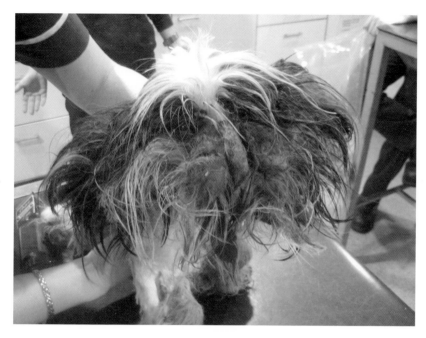

Figure 3.10 For this dog, grooming appears to be very important. (Courtesy of RSPCA Bristol.)

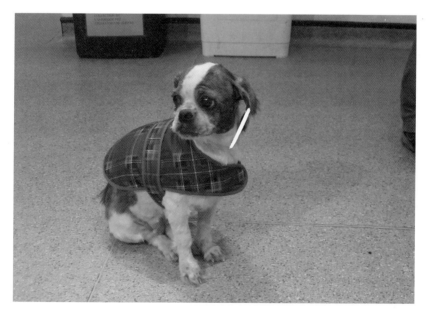

Figure 3.11 Same dog as in Figure 3.9. Grooming is not an urgent need, but presumably it remains as important insofar as it is needed to avoid the dog's previous situation. (Courtesy of RSPCA Bristol.)

always need to be fulfilled before higher ones can be. Humans may deliberately prioritise higher goals – the starved humans in Keys *et al.* (1950) study were conscientious objectors. Indeed, less basic inputs sometimes help to fulfil more basic needs, for example pleasure may improve animals' health and ability to cope with challenge and stress (Lyubomirsky *et al.* 2005). It is probably impossible to place all causes or feelings in strict hierarchies.

3.8 Quantitative Welfare Evaluation

An alternative approach is to try to numerically quantify welfare states. This sounds ambitious but, as we shall see in Chapter 4, quantification can be very useful in making treatment choices. Repeating the same quantitative methods can also be useful to assess changes in welfare state or quality-of-life over time (e.g. Graham *et al.* 2002).

The simplest way to quantify welfare is to ask the owner to give a *gut-feeling* score – or to do it oneself. Unsurprisingly, some owners can find this difficult (Craven *et al.* 2004). One way to make it easier is to use partly qualitative terms, for example defining "1" as "could not be worse" and "10" as "could not be better" (Tzannes *et al.* 2008) or describing the ends of the scale as per the questions in Figure 3.9. But such unstructured quantification is as non-transparent as qualitative methods, and can make discussions harder.

When assessment methods are to be used by many people, they need to aggregate the differing opinions. In some cases, it is possible to ask lots of people in the hope that their errors will cancel each other out, and that their opinions will be normally distributed around the truth. This is what Holton and colleagues did to create the Glasgow Pain Scale (Holton *et al.* 2001). In other cases, disagreements can be minimised by breaking the overall assessment into smaller, more objective *assessment building blocks* and formalising the aggregation process. This is what is done in risk assessment methods (e.g. EFSA 2005, 2006). Ideally, welfare assessment methods should aim at obtaining a consensus between assessors in order to utilise the insights of each. This can be done through a division of labour, with each assessor providing appropriate information for different building blocks (e.g. the veterinary professional about pathological causes and the owner about behaviours at home). Alternatively, consensus may be obtained by discussion, perhaps using formal methods, such as *Delphi approaches* that involve several rounds of formal discussion.

One way to break down the evaluations is to use pre-structured frameworks that add different scores into an overall quantitative welfare score. Aggregative methods can summate the scores of every feeling's valence × intensity × duration × frequency. For example, if an animal experiences pleasure of intensity 3/10 for 2 hours twice, then this generates a score of $(+1) \times (0.3) \times (2) \times (2) = +1.2$ units. If an

Table 3.6 Domains for scoring (adapted from Morton 2007).

Category	Symptoms of positive welfare (score 0 to +2)	Symptoms of negative welfare (score 0 to –4)
Behaviour	Normal activity for individual/species Energetic and relaxed as appropriate	Increased sleep, inactivity Reduced mobility, lameness Abnormal behaviours
Appearance and posture	Alert and confident appearance Appropriate posture	Stance, sunken/dull eyes, staring coat
Appetite	Good, normal appetite Likes treats	Altered eating pattern Reduced body condition Taking longer to finish meal
Provoked behaviours	Exploration and interaction with objects Interacts amicably or plays with others	Specific responses, e.g. pain behaviours Change in temperament Aggression
Health	No clinical symptoms of disease	Specific pathological symptoms
Resources	Freedom to make choices (e.g. untethered) Control over its environment	Excessive defence of resources Fear behaviours towards environment

animal experiences pain of intensity 3/10 for 3 hours once, this scores $(-1) \times (0.3) \times (3) \times (1) = -0.9$ units. If an animal experiences both, then this scores $(+1.2) + (-0.9) = +0.3$ units. This can be simplified by summating quality-of-life scores for given periods of time (e.g. for each day). Ultimately, these scores rely on observable measures of inputs and symptoms. So clinicians could instead quantify and summate the scores of multiple inputs and symptoms, using a system such as the one suggested in Table 3.6 or in the further reading.

Quantitative methods have to work out how to score feelings (or causes and symptoms) on a single comparable scale. For example, they need to address whether three days of pruritus of score 4/10 is worse than two days of pain of Obel lameness score 2/5. Ideally, the score for each input and symptom should be weighted in terms of its potency in causing or signifying feelings, and its specificity and sensitivity in the relevant context. This weighting can be complicated, since the potency, specificity and sensitivity of each may vary depending on their intensity and what other inputs and symptoms are observed.

For assessing the welfare of a herd or group, one can multiply the intensity, duration and frequency by the number of animals affected to give a total score for the herd. This aggregation can be based on the feelings of the average animal, but they should also consider variations between individuals and the effects on outlier individuals at either end of a normal distribution curve.

These questions are about how your dog's life could be made even better.				
Please think when changing your dog's lifestyle would improve their quality of life.				
Please circle your answer.				
1. Environment (where your dog spends most of its time)				
Do you think changing your dog's bed area would improve their life?	**Not at all**	**A little**	**A lot**	**Completely**
2. Exercise and activities (your dog's walks – where, when, how often, how long and how much freedom)				
Do you think changing your dog's exercise regime would improve their life?	**Not at all**	**A little**	**A lot**	**Completely**
3. Diet (what, when and where your dog eats and drinks)				
Do you think changing your dog's diet would improve their life?	**Not at all**	**A little**	**A lot**	**Completely**
4. Mental stimulation (your dog's play, training and toys)				
Do you think changing your dog's opportunities for mental stimulation would improve their life?	**Not at all**	**A little**	**A lot**	**Completely**
5. Companionship with humans				
Do you think changing your dog's human company would improve their life?	**Not at all**	**A little**	**A lot**	**Completely**
6. Companionship with other dogs				
Do you think changing your dog's company with other dogs would improve their life?	**Not at all**	**A little**	**A lot**	**Completely**

Figure 3.12 Questionnaire to assess owners' assessment of lifestyle changes. (Adapted from Mullan and Main 2007.)

3.9 Future Welfare Evaluation

Most decisions in practice are ultimately based not on assessments of animals' *previous* welfare, but on assessments of their *future* welfare, for example predicting the outcomes of different treatment options. Such prospective assessments are even more complicated than assessments of an animal's previous or current welfare. They require multiple evaluations when there are several treatment options or possible outcome, including disease progression, response to treatment, likely longevity, possible complications, further sequelae, risks of new diseases or accidents and euthanasia. Future assessments cannot simply observe the animal but rely on the clinician's ability to prophesy what possibilities could happen and the likelihood of each possibility.

One can ask owners how they think various changes would affect the animal, as in Figure 3.12. We could qualitatively list the pros and cons of each option. Tables 3.7 and 3.8 show an example of harms, risks and benefits for amputation versus a limb-sparing operation and chemotherapy versus no chemotherapy for canine distal limb osteosarcoma. Such lists can be helpful to frame discussions with owners, but they do not obviously help to weigh up the relative importance of each pro and con.

We could also quantitatively evaluate treatments by extending the mathematical formula of valence, intensity, duration, frequency and number to also include probability. For example, if a surgical procedure gives a 20% chance of a month of

Table 3.7 Benefits, certain harms and risks for leg amputation versus limb-sparing surgery for canine distal limb osteosarcoma.

	Amputation	**Limb-sparing surgery**
Benefits	• Good pain-relief (no leg) • Cheaper • Minimal surgical aftercare (e.g. visits to vet or rest)	• Full or good use of leg
Expected harms	• Need to adapt to loss of leg • Pain if arthritis in other leg	• Probably more painful • Relatively intense aftercare, e.g. dressing changes • Foot swelling
Risks	• Anaesthetic risk (death) • Femoral arterial bleed (death) • Phantom limb syndrome? • (Drug reactions, e.g. to analgesics)	• Infection • Implant failure • Local recurrence • Flexure contracture • (May then require amputation) • (Drug reactions, e.g. to analgesics)

Table 3.8 Benefits, certain harms and risks for chemotherapy versus no chemotherapy for canine distal limb osteosarcoma.

	No chemotherapy	Chemotherapy
Benefits	• Fewer visits to vet or rest • Cheaper	• Longer expected survival time
Expected harms		• Nausea • Repeated visits for blood tests and chemotherapy
Risks	• Likely sooner metastasis	• (Drug reactions, e.g. to analgesics) • Chemotherapy risks, e.g. kidney or heart muscle toxicity, blood problems and infections

severe pain (score −2 units) but an 80% chance of a month of moderate happiness (score +1 units), then the overall score for surgery is $(0.20) \times (-2) + (0.80) \times (+1) = +0.8$. This approach is reminiscent of a very influential theory in human economics called "*expected* utility theory", which bases assessments on mathematical calculations of predicted mental welfare. The idea was proposed in the eighteenth century by economists such as Bernoulli (1738) and Jevons (1871) and, perhaps surprisingly, such mathematical models have proven quite accurate in predicting peoples' thinking (Nickerson 2008).

Our predictions can be based either on extrapolating general knowledge (e.g. scientific data) to the individual or on extrapolating historical information about the individual (e.g. previous responses to treatment) to the future. However, we cannot objectively predict probabilities when we lack an evidence base or are unclear how it applies to the specific patient. In such cases, a different approach is suggested by a more recent development in economics called "*subjective* expected utility theory" (Savage 1954). Instead of using probabilities, decision-makers can score their *confidence* in their predictions. As the name suggests, using clinician confidence approach is more subjective than using recorded probabilities, and may be more prone to biases. Nevertheless, subjective expected utility predictions are suitable for quantitative methods when scientific evidence of probabilities is unavailable.

Because future welfare evaluations are prospective, whether an evaluation is correct is *not* a matter of what outcomes actually happen. For example, a veterinary professional may judge that analgesia is beneficial for calves they are disbudding. If one calf suffers a reaction to an analgesic, this does not mean that the decision to give analgesia to that calf was wrong. Put another way, one can make the right decision and then have *bad welfare luck*.

Summary and key recommendations

- Animal welfare assessment is vital for veterinary practice, whether it is done informally or formally. Veterinary surgeons, nurses and owners can contribute valuable insights to joint assessment.
- Screening assessment involves two steps of information and interpretation to identify issues. Information from history-taking, clinical examination and further tests can look at causes and symptoms of pathological and other welfare issues. Obtaining information can cause iatrogenic harms. Clinical measures seem more objective, but this is often illusory, since such measures still need to be interpreted. Interpretation should focus on the individual patient, using processes of empathy or egomorphism, combined with induction or hypothetico-deduction.
- Gauging animal welfare involves a further step of evaluation to help make decisions. Qualitative Welfare Evaluation can assess welfare as *bad*, *worse* or whether *needs* are fulfilled. Such intuitive judgements are common but controversial. Quantitative Welfare Evaluation can generate numerical scores, for example considering feelings' valence × intensity × duration × frequency for all feelings of all animals. Quantitative Welfare Evaluation is also controversial but more transparent.
- Future Welfare Evaluation involves making predictions based on probability or confidence. Such prospective assessments may be correct even if unlikely outcomes occur due to *bad welfare luck*.

Selected further reading

General approaches to assessing behaviour are given by Martin and Bateson (2007), more background information by McGreevy (2004), Hosey *et al.* (2009) and Houpt (2011) and insights into its underreporting by Bradshaw *et al.* (2002), APBC (2005) and Blackwell *et al.* (2005). Lists of normal parameters for various populations are given by Lumsden *et al.* (1980), Tadich *et al.* (1997) and Gul *et al.* (2007). General references for assessing animal welfare include Spinelli and Markowitz (1987) and CAWC (2009); McMillan 2003 and Yeates and Main (2009) are specifically related to veterinary practice.

Qualitative empathetic interpretations are discussed by Wemelsfelder (1997), and Maslow's hierarchy by Maslow (1943) and Curtis (1983). Needs and psychological needs are discussed by Hurnik and Lehman (1988), Jensen and Toates (1993), Broom (1999) and Young (1999) regarding animals and by Lightfoot (1995), Culyer (1998) and Asadi-Lari *et al.* (2003) regarding human medicine. There are many needs-based welfare assessment frameworks for farm animals (e.g. Bracke *et al.* 1999; Bartussek 2001; Capdeville & Veissier 2001), for rodents (e.g. Balcombe 2006), chickens (e.g. Weeks & Nichol 2006), horses (Zeeb 1981) and humans (e.g. Bengtsson-Tops & Hansson 1999; Griffiths *et al.* 2007).

Scales are given for pain in horses (e.g. Bussieres *et al.* 2008), dogs (e.g. Holton *et al.* 2001; Wiseman-Orr *et al.* 2004, 2006; Hellyer *et al.* 2007; Reid *et al.* 2007) and cats (e.g. Brondani *et al.* 2011) for pruritus (e.g. Ahlstrom *et al.* 2009; Favrot *et al.* 2010); for lameness and limb function (e.g. Hudson *et al.* 2004; Robinson *et al.* 2007); body condition scores (e.g. Zanella *et al.* 2003; German 2006, German *et al.* 2007); fractures (e.g. Aron *et al.* 1995); disseminated intravascular coagulation (e.g. Winberg *et al.* 2010) and for breed-related disease severity (e.g. Asher *et al.* 2010). More general scores for health-related quality-of-life are given for dogs (e.g. Wojciechowska & Hewson 2005), cats (Hartmann & Kuffer 1998) and pigs (Wiseman-Orr *et al.* 2011a,b). Measuring health in human medicine is discussed by Bowling (2005).

The intensity, duration and numbers approach is discussed for wild animals by Kirkwood *et al.* (1994). Examples of quantitative approaches to herd assessment are reported for farm animal assessments (e.g. Main *et al.* 2003; Whay *et al.* 2003; Müller-Graf *et al.* 2008), companion animals (e.g. Wojciechowska *et al.* 2005; Morton 2007), zoo animals (e.g. Föllmi *et al.* 2007) and laboratory animals (Wolfensohn & Honess 2007). Risk assessment methodologies are described by Müller-Graf *et al.* (2008). The EU Welfare Quality Project is a recent major attempt to generate a quantitative assessment method for multiple animals, described by Botreau *et al.* (2009). *Expected utility theory* is classically discussed by von Neumann and Morgenstern (1944).

Disagreements between assessors are evidenced by, for example, Chang and Yeh (2005), and collaboration by Higashi *et al.* (2005) and Varni *et al.* (2007). Delphi approaches are described by Main *et al.* (2003), Whay *et al.* (2003) and Collins *et al.* (2009). The website www.usability.gov gives guidelines for web-based tool design, as do the journals *Quality of Life Research* and *Health and Quality of Life Outcomes*.

Clinical Choices

4

4.1 Welfare-Focused Choices

Having made an assessment of an animal's welfare, especially its future welfare, the next step is to decide what to do with that information (Figure 4.1). There are many different ways we can make choices in veterinary practice. Like owners, we can make choices using our emotions. As discussed in Chapter 2, such emotions can be very useful, especially when time is short and one knows the animal well. But they can bias our decision-making, for example by focusing on ourselves (e.g. whether we will help or harm) rather than the animal (e.g. whether the patient will improve or worsen). This can lead to an *intervention bias*, where we prefer options that improve welfare through our action rather than inaction (e.g. treating conditions that would improve on their own or providing prophylactic treatment for rare conditions).

Decisions vary in importance. There are *big deals* and there are *little matters* (Figure 4.2). The time spent on a decision should be proportionate to its importance (Audi 2006). It is easy to magnify little decisions into great agonies of choice, or to repeatedly question one's decisions. All treatment decisions need some thought, even decisions to book revisits or to perform a diagnostic test, but some decisions can be made more efficiently, or followed and only occasionally reviewed. It is equally easy to make big decisions without sufficient respect for the magnitude of that decision.

Our decisions may be improved by using structured methods that make our deliberations more rational, unbiased and transparent. Sometimes we can make

Animal Welfare in Veterinary Practice, First Edition. James Yeates.
© 2013 Universities Federation for Animal Welfare. Published 2013 by Blackwell Publishing Ltd.

Step of decision making process	Example of step for a euthanasia decision
CHOICE-MAKING PROCESS	Owner reflects on the matter and discusses it with spouse, deciding to euthanase the dog soon
AVAILABLE OPTION CHOSEN	The veterinarian refuses to provide unreasonable treatment options so the dog is immediately euthanased

Figure 4.1   Model of choice-making by veterinary professionals.

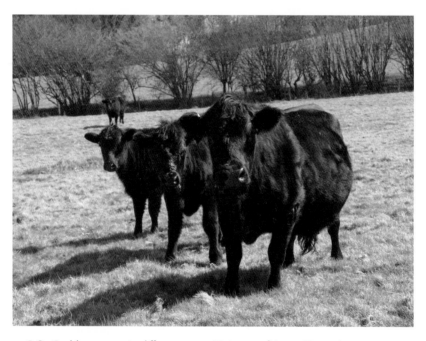

Figure 4.2   Problems come in different sizes. (Courtesy of James Yeates.)

decisions using fixed and absolute rules. For example, one might consider that one should never perform a surgical operation for purely cosmetic reasons, provide non-emergency treatment without valid consent or break the law. However, we need other methods to make decisions where such rules do not decide our choices.

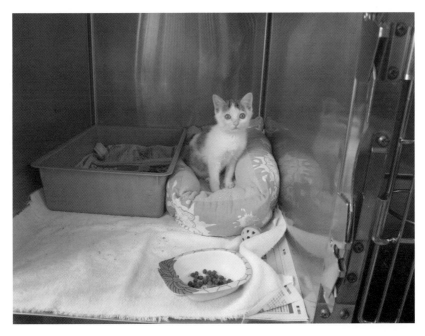

Figure 4.3 Animals may have very different experiences of treatment to human patients. (Courtesy of SPCA Hong Kong.)

Sometimes we can refer to *gold standard* treatments described in textbooks. However, textbook advice is like scientific findings in that it needs to be adapted to individual clients. There is no such thing as *best practice* in the sense of a treatment that should always be done. What is right for each patient is a *bespoke practice* that fits with the particular animal's individual personality, circumstances and takes into account the relevant owner-based, financial and other constraints. (Remembering this may help practitioners to feel less frustrated or guilty for providing such treatments – they are best for this case, and this more complex problem-solving is part of the skill of veterinary practice.)

In some cases we might respect our clients' wishes, as human doctors do. However, veterinary professionals should not unthinkingly leave decisions to clients, nor simply transpose decisions from human medicine. Human patients are very different to animal patients, and veterinary professionals' duties are very different to human medical professionals'. Applying human treatment choices is a form of anthropomorphism and should be done critically by considering human–non-human differences. Humans may have very different biology, pathology, pharmacology, psychology and experience of treatment. Humans may want to see their grandchild's wedding, feel guilty for taking up resources, fear the afterlife, understand treatment, consider their life as *sacred* and have *human dignity*, all of which may not apply to animals (Figure 4.3). Similar considerations guard against egomorphically choosing the option you would want if you were the patient. It is often better to ignore what is good for humans and instead to choose veterinary treatments based on more basic evaluations and clinical reasoning.

Ideally, clinical choices should be based on future welfare evaluations, by choosing the option with the best balance of *costs* and *benefits*. This cost–benefit analysis method can consider one stakeholder or several. Some decisions concern only individuals (discussed in Section 4.2), others concern multiple animals (Sections 4.3 and 4.4) and others concern animals and humans (Sections 4.5, 4.6, 4.7 and 4.8). Each of these involves increasingly wider considerations and decision-making.

THE ANIMALS

4.2 Individual Patients

Treatments may affect animals' welfare in many different ways. They may directly prevent feelings (e.g. analgesia or anxiolytics) or cause them (e.g. nausea or dysphoria). They may avoid the causes of feelings (e.g. curative medications), mask their symptoms (e.g. some uses of sedatives) or increase the risk factors for such causes (e.g. through nephrotoxicity or surgical lesions). They may also extend life or shorten it (e.g. through deliberate euthanasia or through risky procedures).

There is no categorical list of what treatments are in patients' interests. Bespoke practice will therefore vary for different patients. Medications can be contraindicated by allergies or concomitant diseases. Hospitalisation or frequent visits can be contraindicated by severe vet-fear. Long courses of medication or risky procedures may be contraindicated by anticipated owner non-compliance, inability to fund future treatment for complications or likely unwillingness to consent to later euthanasia. Breed, lifestyle and human–animal relationships mean different animals have varying background risks of disease or expected lifespans. The right treatment for each case depends on the individual animal and its particular circumstances.

In general terms, there are two types of mistreatment (Figure 4.4). *Undertreatment* is where animals do not get treatments that could be provided and that would be in their interests. *Overtreatment* is where animals get any treatment that is not in their interests, compared to more conservative options such as (a) no treatment or (b) euthanasia. It is impossible to give a definitive list of overtreatments or under-treatments, but higher risk treatments that may be more likely to constitute overtreatment are suggested in Table 4.1.

Often, mistreatment involves both undertreatment and overtreatment. If a patient receives an ineffective antibiotic, then it both lacks a worthwhile

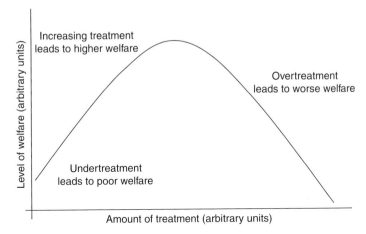

Figure 4.4 Two types of mistreatment: undertreatment and overtreatment.

Table 4.1 Categories of overtreatment and examples that may be overtreatment for some individuals (after Yeates 2010b).

Comparison	*Acute*	*Chronic*
More conservative treatment	Performance-enhancing or cosmetic surgery	Chemotherapy for "surgical tumour"
		Excessive prophylaxis
	Removal of benign tumour	Unnecessary disease monitoring
Euthanasia	Large-scale tissue resection (other than limb)	Perpetuation of life of suffering patient
		Poorly tolerated chemotherapy
	Hoisting a long-term cast horse or downer cow	Long-term hospitalisation of wild animal

treatment and receives a potentially harmful drug. Similarly, surgery without adequate analgesia may be both undertreatment insofar as the animal does not receive required painkillers and overtreatment insofar as the animal may be better off without the highly painful surgery.

Choosing the bespoke treatment should be based on evaluations of the patient's future welfare for each treatment option, including no treatment and euthanasia. The option that is evaluated as best is the one that should be prioritised. This evaluation may be based on qualitative evaluations, such as criteria like *extreme suffering* (which is not easily defined), hierarchies or binary criteria. Such methods may be especially useful for planning and communication with owners, as they are easy to understand and can set objective thresholds. For example, binary methods work well when it is clear what each change will mean – for example, that a change in any sole parameter is sufficient to prescribe euthanasia. If this is not clear, and

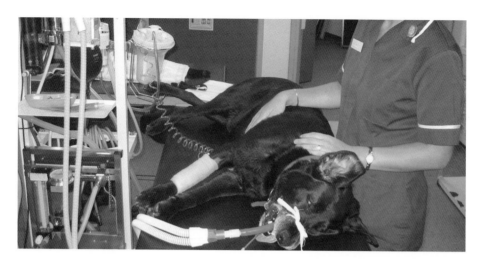

Figure 4.5 Anaesthesia itself does not involve feelings, and hence can be given neutral value in quantitative methods (although the feelings during induction and recovery do involve feelings that should be considered). (Courtesy of RSPCA Bristol.)

some parameters worsen and others improve, then we still need to make a judgement about which are more important.

Qualitative methods are not good at taking risks into account. For example, we may think a small risk of extreme suffering or failing to satisfy a vital need does not outweigh a high probability of achieving a better outcome (otherwise this would rule out any non-life-saving treatments or euthanasia). Risk is more easily handled by quantitative methods which consider the severity, duration, frequency and likelihood of pleasant and unpleasant feelings that will occur in the different possible outcomes for each option. For example, pleasant life may have positive value, suffering a negative value and the absence of feelings such as anaesthesia a neutral value (Figure 4.5). Quantitative decision-making can be based on thresholds applied to the quantitative assessments discussed in Section 3.7. For example, Table 4.2 suggests some decision-making thresholds based on Table 3.6.

Because quantitative methods involve a consideration of the *duration* of future feelings, they need to consider the animal's expected longevity and welfare for each option, so quality-of-life and quantity-of-life can be balanced. One approach is to consider extended life as being worth achieving or avoiding based on the expected quality-of-life (FAWC 2009; Yeates 2011b, 2012b). Animals may be kept alive if their future life is expected to involve good feelings that outweigh the negative feelings, i.e. they have a *life-worth-living*. Animals should be euthanased if death is in the animal's interests (Yeates 2010c). Death is in an animal's interests when their future life is expected to involve more suffering than enjoyment, i.e. they have a *life-worth-avoiding* (Wathes 2010; Yeates 2011b). This means that *quantity-of-life*

Table 4.2 Guide to interpreting overall positive and negative summated scores (adapted from Morton 2007).

Score	Interpretation	Prescription
+5 to +11	Has a life-worth-living	Major adjustments should be avoided
0 to +5		Major adjustments not warranted, but would benefit from some changes
–7 to 0	Has a life-worth-avoiding	QOL should be improved immediately (e.g. within 1 week)
–8 to –15		Major changes needed, alongside regular review of treatment and prognosis
–16 to –24		Euthanasia mandated unless high chance of improvement within 3 days

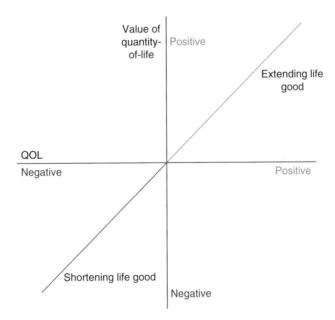

Figure 4.6 The value of quantity-of-life based on the quality-of-life experienced.

is not a separate value to quality-of-life, but that the value of quantity-of-life depends entirely on the animal's expected quality-of-life (Figure 4.6).

Veterinary professionals should work out whether a patient's life would be worth living or worth avoiding when one's options include euthanasia, a life-saving treatment (e.g. resuscitation) or an intervention that could constitute overtreatment. But how do we work out whether a life is worth living or avoiding

---

Box 4.1   Formula for Calculating Quality-Adjusted-Life-Years (QALYs), Quality-Adjusted-Life-Months (QALMs) and Quality-Adjusted-Life-Periods (QALPs) from quality of life (QOL) and lifespan assessments.

QALYs for Option 1 = average expected QOL (out of 1) × average expected lifespan (years)

QALMs for Option 1 = average expected QOL (out of 1) × average expected lifespan (months)

QALPs for Option 1 = (severity × duration × probability of Outcome 1) + ... + (severity × duration × probability of Outcome N)

---

if it involves a mixture of periods of good and bad welfare? And what about comparing between treatments that both lead to a life-worth-living but vary in the lifespan and quality-of-life? In these cases, a more complex method to balance quality-of-life and quantity-of-life is required.

The idea of quality-adjusted-life-years (QALYs) is used in human medicine to decide how to allocate funds for different treatments for different people, but we can also use them to decide between treatments for an individual patient. The basic idea is that each treatment option is rated in terms of the longevity that it is expected to provide multiplied by the overall quality-of-life that the treatment would provide. In human QALY calculations, quality-of-life is usually rated as "1" when the patient is completely healthy and poorer quality lives are scored between 0 and 1 (Harris 1987). Veterinary practitioners might use shorter periods than years – such as *quality-adjusted-life-months* (QALMs). These are calculated using the formula in Box 4.1. So, for example, 6 months with perfect welfare would score $6 \times 1 = 6$ QALMs, whereas 1 year with quality-of-life of score 0.3 would score $12 \times 0.3 = 4$ QALMs. The first treatment would therefore be chosen.

This concept can fit with the ideas of a life-worth-living and a life-worth-avoiding, by considering using negative quality-of-life scores. Medical assessments usually consider human life to always have positive value (Kaplan *et al.* 2007), but we can score animal's lives-worth-avoiding as less than 0. Death is rated as 0, not because being dead prevents any feelings, but simply because it involves 0 life years (and 0 times any quality-of-life score equals 0).

Of course, animals' lives are not always of unvarying quality-of-life. Most treatments provide a number of periods in which animals may experience a different quality-of-life. Animals' lives are also not entirely predictable. Most treatments provide a number of *risks* of possible longevity and quality-of-life. Ultimately, this concept can be made even more sophisticated by working out the quality-of-life for each of the different periods of life that each treatment would provide and the probability that each period will occur. These can be multiplied to create an overall

Box 4.2   Steps for Calculating QALPs.

1. Identify all possible treatment options
2. Identify all the possible outcomes for each option
3. Assess the quality-of-life and duration of each outcome
4. Assess the probability of each outcome occurring
5. Calculate an outcome score for each outcome by multiplying the expected quality-of-life × duration × probability
6. Aggregate the scores of each possible outcome multiplied by its probability

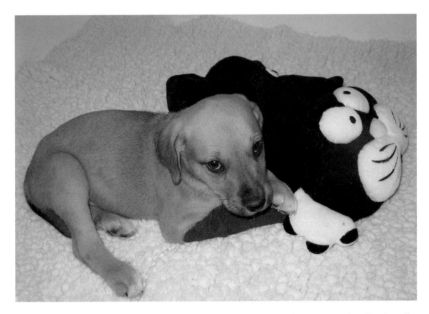

Figure 4.7 In quantitative methods like QALYs, the age of an animal will alter their life expectancy. (Courtesy of RSPCA Bristol.)

qualitative assessment, which we might call *quality-adjusted-life-periods* (QALPs), using the steps described in Box 4.2. These effectively lead to the formula in Box 4.1.

Using QALYs have disadvantages. It has certain inherent biases, such as preferring life-saving treatments for younger animals, with which not everyone may agree (Figure 4.7). The calculations may be difficult and counter-intuitive and may seem coldly uncaring, especially for *life and death* decisions. The conclusions may conflict with more intuitive clinical decisions and may be ignored. This means that, until the method has been developed and validated, QALYs would be used best as a device to assist reflective decision-making but not to definitively determine treatment choices.

4.3 Decisions Affecting Multiple Patients

In many cases, we have to consider multiple animals, such as a whole flock or herd, or when transplanting blood or kidneys from one animal to another, or when considering practising or experimenting on our patients.

Some cases are simple because one option is in every animal's interests. Some treatments may improve every animal's welfare, for example, better fly control and dagging to avoid the need for tail-docking may benefit every lamb. Other treatments may be worthwhile for every animal, even if they only benefit some animals and even harm others; for example, vaccinating a flock may cause some vaccination reactions but is still indicated for each individual. Similarly, one may reduce post-ovariohysterectomy haemorrhage rates by double-ligating ovarian vessels, but the slower surgery time may increase anaesthetic risks, such as post-anaesthetic dysphoria or post-operative mortality. If the risks of haemorrhage outweigh the anaesthetic risks, then double-ligation is in the interests of each individual patient, even though some unlucky patients are harmed.

Other cases are more complicated because they involve ignoring or harming some animals in order to benefit others. For example, one might have to decide whether to kill a few members of a herd for post-mortem, isolate an individual to prevent infection or de-horn steers or tooth-clip piglets to prevent them harming others.

For these cases, veterinary professionals may use quantitative methods to aggregate the welfare of all animals involved. For example, tail-docking causes sheep pain and distress but may prevent a proportion of the sheep suffering from fly-strike. In the case given in Box 4.3, the calculation suggests the decision should be not to tail-dock the lambs. This decision is highly case-specific – for example, it would suggest that tail-docking should be done if the expected incidence of fly-strike in non-tail-docked lambs increased from 4% to 5%. So the method could lead to different decisions in other situations, e.g. for store lambs, November lambing, easy-care lambs, for mulesing instead of tail-docking, if fly-struck lambs were euthanased earlier, etc.

An alternative approach is to use a hierarchical method that prioritises certain outcomes over others. One hierarchical method is to use a *bottom-up rule* to choose whatever option improves the welfare of the worst off. Another hierarchical method is a *rights-based rule* to reject any option that causes any animal to have welfare below a certain level, for example a life-worth-avoiding. For example, in the tail-docking decision in Box 4.3, we might think that avoiding any animal experiencing the catastrophic event of fly-strike is more important than preventing minor pain and distress (even in a larger number of animals). This would suggest we should subject all animals to tail-docking (even if only 1% of the flock would be expected to get fly-strike).

In practice, one may choose to use a combination of hierarchical and quantitative approaches. One may think that one should avoid certain severe harms to any

Box 4.3   QALYs-based decision-making for tail-docking a flock of lambs.

Case:	
Number of animals	100
Average life expectancy	150 days

Assessments:

Mutilations – cause pain and distress

Average intensity score	−5
(see Kent et al. 1993; Jongman *et al.* 2000)	
Average duration	1 day
(see Shutt *et al.* 1987; Peers *et al.* 2002;	
Thornton & Waterman-Pearson 2002)	
Numbers whole flock, i.e. 100 lambs	

Fly-strike – distress and malaise

Average intensity score	−10
(see Colditz et al. 2005; Phillips 2009)	
Average duration	10 days
(Lee and Fisher 2007)	
Numbers expected 4% flock, i.e. 4 lambs	

Normal life with/without tail

Average score	+1
Average life until flystrike	140 days

QALY scores

Mutilations	[procedure] + [good life]	
	[−5 × 1 days × 100] + [1 × 149 days × 100])	
Total		= 14 400
Risking fly-strike	[good life] + [disease]	
Affected:	[1 × 140 days x 4] + [−10 × 10 days × 4]	
Unaffected:	[1 × 150 days × 96]	
Total		=14 560

individual (e.g. substantial suffering), but that more minor harms can be balanced across individuals using quantitative methods.

4.4 Decisions Also Affecting Non-Patient Animals

Often treatments affect both patients and non-patient animals. Some treatments are win-win. Vaccination not only helps an individual, but also contributes to population immunity through vaccination of individuals. Novel therapies can be helpful to the individual and also progress veterinary medicine. Neutering can provide health benefits and facilitate group housing of gregarious species (e.g. rabbits). Unfortunately, other treatments create *welfare dilemmas*.

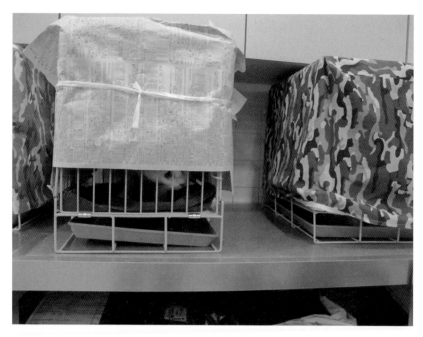

Figure 4.8 Trap-Neuter-Return programmes cause unpleasant experiences for individuals, but benefit other animals. (Courtesy of SPCA Hong Kong.)

Some treatments create welfare dilemmas because they benefit the patient but harm other animals. Surgical interventions may perpetuate breed-related conditions. Prescribing mutilations or antibiotics may support the continued use of imperfect husbandry conditions. Releasing wild animals may affect local populations. Recommending chicken as a bland diet may lead to increased sales of chicken raised in poor welfare standards. Using many pharmaceuticals perpetuates the use of laboratory animals in research, development and testing.

Other treatments create welfare dilemmas because they harm the patient to benefit others. Killing an aggressive dog or a cat infected with feline leukaemia virus (FeLV) may prevent it disseminating the disease or hurting others. Risky clinical trials may jeopardise the individual's welfare but can improve veterinary techniques. These cases also place veterinary professionals in a dilemma. Neutering, as in Trap-Neuter-Return (TNR) programmes, may help population control but may not necessarily benefit all the animals neutered (Figure 4.8).

One solution to such welfare dilemmas is to consider all animals' interests equally, for example by calculating the QALMs for all affected animals. This approach has dangerous implications; for example, it would justify experimenting on one's patients in order to develop treatments for other animals. An opposite approach would be to consider only our patients. This approach has dangerous implications; for example, it would justify choices like releasing FeLV positive cats or embezzling owners' money to subsidise pro bono work on unowned animals.

One middle ground is the 'avoiding harm approach': to consider that (a) veterinary professionals may benefit our patients without harming other animals, (b) we may not harm our patients to benefit other animals and (c) we may harm our patients if this is necessary to avoid them harming other animals. This means we can provide any treatment to our patients that do not harm other animals, and also we can isolate or euthanase animals if this could lead to them infecting many other animals. It also means we should not deliberately experiment on our patients, although deriving information from cases is a legitimate side effect.

Another approach is for veterinary professionals to proactively take steps to remedy the causes of dilemmas, in order to compensate for the harms they cause to other animals through helping their patients. For example, where veterinary surgeons feel obliged to perform elective caesarians without spaying, and thereby help perpetuate breed-related conditions, they could actively work with or lobby breeding clubs or government to improve standards. Such *welfare offsetting* may help a veterinary professional to maintain a positive welfare account.

THE HUMANS

4.5 Oneself

Often clinicians are affected by their own concerns and interests. Treatment decisions can benefit veterinary professionals in several ways (Box 4.4). While this book focuses on welfare-focused rather than vet-focused practice, concern for oneself can legitimately serve as a constraint or side effect of providing treatment.

Some vet-focused motivations are *ego-focused*. Veterinary professionals may enjoy the success of curing a patient, performing a heroic surgery, gaining knowledge through case-based learning, completing a specialist qualification or finding a diagnosis. Others may feel ignorance to be personally unpleasant or euthanasia to be a personal failure. From a welfare perspective, such ego-focused practice is illegitimate. Such personal benefits are legitimate *side effects* of welfare-focused treatment but should not be the aim of practice. They should never cause a veterinary professional to overtreat a patient.

One specific example of an ego-focused concern is the motivation to obtaining a diagnosis. Diagnoses have indirect value when they help to make informed treatment choices. But wanting a diagnosis for its own good is *diagnosis fetishism*, which can lead to overtreatment. Diagnoses should be sought only if doing so provides valuable information and is worth the iatrogenic harms of the procedures needed to obtain it (Figure 4.9). A diagnosis may not be valuable if, for example, the treatment would be the same, or if the owner does not have sufficient funds to provide treatment after a diagnosis is reached (including if the investigation needed to reach a diagnosis would use up the insurance limit on the owner's policy).

Box 4.4   Elements of vet-focused practice.

Ego-focused practice

- Satisfying intellectual curiosity (e.g. diagnosis fetishism)
- Successfully "solving" a case
- Keeping an animal alive
- Saving an animal that others had given up on
- Proving "pessimists" wrong
- Passing an examination which requires a certain number of procedures to have been conducted
- Building a professional reputation
- Self-perception as a "pioneer"
- Feeling "heroic"

Emotion-focused practice

- Satisfaction of doing good
- Avoiding guilt
- Job satisfaction

Money-focused practice

- Covering costs
- Increasing profit
- Improving client relationships
- Improving public relations

Law-focused practice

- Avoid litigation
- Avoid criminal proceedings

A subtler example of an ego-focused concern is the motivation to feel good about having personally helped a patient. This concern can motivate us to help our patients, but it can create a bias towards providing overtreatment, for example if animals would otherwise improve on their own. Conversely, another ego-focused motivation is to avoid feeling bad for having harmed a patient. This motivation can help to highlight possible iatrogenic harms, but it can also create a bias towards undertreatment, for example by leaving animals to die by natural processes.

Other vet-focused motivations are *law-focused*. Veterinary professionals may fear prosecution for criminal offences (e.g. theft or destruction of property for killing), litigation (e.g. negligence) or disciplinary proceedings (e.g. professional misconduct). Obeying the law provides a legitimate *constraint* on what treatment options are available to the veterinary professional. Legal duties can therefore

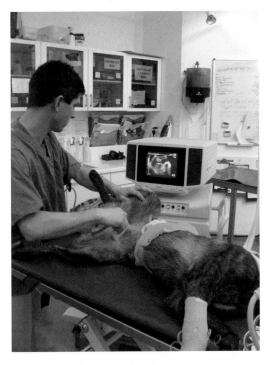

Figure 4.9 A diagnosis is worthwhile only when the information's value to the patient outweighs the iatrogenic harms of the procedures. (Courtesy of RSPCA Bristol.)

legitimise undertreatment (e.g. not treating an animal against the owner's wishes). However, veterinary professionals should not be overly concerned about possible legal challenges. Being sued risks causing a financial loss (for which many professionals are insured), and a clinician may feel this risk is worth taking to improve an animal's welfare. Plus, both criminal and civil law often allow animal welfare concerns to provide a legitimate defence.

One specific example of a law-focused motivation is the temptation to offer all options in order to guarantee you have obtained valid informed consent. For example, one may feel that a cast horse or cow needs euthanasia, but one may feel obliged to also mention the option of trying to hoist it. If the owner selects this option, it becomes difficult to then refuse to provide it. It may be better not to offer an unreasonable option at all, or at least to be clear that you would not be prepared to provide it. If one's legal duty is to offer all reasonable options, then not offering *unreasonable* options should be legitimate. Veterinary professionals should offer only reasonable options.

Other vet-focused motivations are *money-focused*. Practices need to cover overheads in order to continue to provide veterinary services and to give veterinary professionals a fair pay for their expertise. Making money involves charging fees, which can lead to undertreatment when owners refuse to pay, and maintaining a client base, which can lead to overtreatment when owners request it. Money-focused concerns can provide another legitimate *constraint* against providing treatment, since practices cannot sustainably provide unlimited subsidised treatment. This constraint means that practices should set and charge reasonable fees that allow them to maintain a service. However, money-focused concerns should not be the aim of veterinary practice. Veterinary professionals should not provide treatment in order to make money, but financial gains may be a legitimate side effect of providing treatment.

In addition, clinicians should keep in mind that, while some people are driven by money, one can sometimes increase one's own welfare more by being altruistic than by being richer. For example, some veterinary practices provide free euthanasia, even out of hours, so that they never risk the feeling of having to leave a suffering animal without offering one option to improve its welfare. Many practices have systems for providing a substantial amount of pro bono treatment, and this can be valuable for improving public relations to clients or referring practices.

In summary, good practice may be *constrained* by satisfying vet-focused motivations, but should never be *construed* as satisfying them and such biases should be avoided or minimised. Vet-focused concerns may sometimes justify undertreatment, but very rarely justify overtreatment. However, practitioners should not be ashamed of the fact that they make money, enjoy their job, learn from their previous cases, maintain good public relations and have not been sued, when these are achieved as a side effect of welfare-focused veterinary work.

4.6 Colleagues

Other vet-focused motivations concern one's colleagues, both within a practice and between practices.

Other vet-focused motivations concern veterinary professionals' employers. Employees may be motivated to benefit their employer, for example through making money. Employers may influence clinical decisions through direct orders, through limiting what equipment or drugs are available or through a subtler cultural influence of "this is how we do things here". Employers' opinions can be useful if they are knowledgeable and experienced practitioners. However, employers are not necessarily experts at welfare assessment and may not make better decisions than employees about the latter's patient. They may also have particular biases, such as motivations towards making money or keeping clients. In some cases, employers are not veterinary professionals, meaning that they do not have the same professional values and accountabilities.

Practitioners should take full responsibility for their own decisions and cannot legitimately transfer their animal welfare account to their employers. Employers' opinions should sometimes be disregarded to achieve animal welfare goals. At the same time, employers should check that they do not place undesirable influence on their employees through cynicism, megalomania, money-focus or arrogance.

Other vet-focused motivations concern one's colleagues. Veterinary profession-als may be concerned about their colleagues' interests, such as job satisfaction, financial rewards, litigation and disciplinary proceedings. Veterinary professionals may also want to obtain colleagues' respect. The opinion of one's peers creates a *social norm* that can affect one's decisions. As with other emotional methods of decision-making, this can provide a useful way to highlight areas of concern. But it may be better to use more reflective and animal-focused motivations.

As one example, veterinary professionals may be tempted to perform a proce-dure because they know that another veterinary professional will otherwise do it. On the one hand, it is unacceptable to provide a treatment merely because other veterinary professionals do so: this argument does not work for overtreatment any more than it does for murder. In fact, refusing can improve welfare by highlighting the ethical controversy to the owner and the other veterinary professional and per-haps by progressing the profession's standards. Refusing also preserves your integ-rity and may avoid you feeling guilty. On the other hand, providing the treatment can be better for the patient if you are more competent or it avoids the animal hav-ing to travel. Such *tactical overtreatment* is not really overtreatment because it is the bespoke treatment for the animal. Overtreatment should not be provided so that the client saves money, or so that you make money instead of the other practice.

The influence of colleagues can be avoided through communication and coordina-tion between colleagues. Informal agreements (e.g. not to destroy a healthy dog) or *standard operating procedures* (SOPs) that prescribe what should be done for par-ticular cases can help. Coordination can help to make treatment decisions consistent and avoids veterinary professionals having erroneous beliefs about what treatments colleagues will provide. Clinicians may then be faced with dilemmas when they think that the bespoke treatment would require breaching a SOP. Clinicians need to be flex-ible in their decision-making where necessary and achieve joint decision-making and valid consent, but consider veterinary professionals should therefore consider deviat-ing from SOPs if, and only if, the particular case provides specific reasons to do so.

4.7 Clients

Another key stakeholder is the human owner. Clients can deliberately put pressure on veterinary professionals to make certain decisions, through coercion or by giv-ing or withholding consent or fees. Clients can unconsciously pressure veterinary professionals who are concerned about client satisfaction or their clients' interests.

At other times, clients' choices do not coincide with what is good for the patient. An owner may want a horse doped to win a race, a problem behaviour stopped by any means, a rehomable animal euthanased for convenience or a suffering animal kept alive. Some veterinary professionals look to balance the interests of the client and patient. One way to balance these is to consider that treatment choices can be con-strained by clients' choices, but not construed as them. Legitimate constraints include where the animal might harm the owner or other humans, for example if it is untreatably aggressive or has a major zoonotic disease. Similarly, the lack of owner consent in non-emergency cases can serve as a legal constraint. But owners' wishes cannot create a mandate to provide treatment, and veterinary professionals are responsible for any treatment we provide. We need to decide what treatments we provide. As for other focuses, benefitting clients can serve as a legitimate side effect of treating patients.

In many cases where owners do not make welfare-focused choices, they are unreasonable owners. It would be better if owners took their animal welfare responsibilities seriously and always wanted to do what was in the interests of their animal. Unfortunately, this is not always the case and the inadequacies of the owner need to be considered when evaluating the best welfare-focused approach. Veterinary professionals are caught in dilemmas between two options.

One option is to "keep your hands clean". One can decide what should be done in an ideal world, even if this choice is not best for the individual patient. This might involve refusing to provide certain treatments in any circumstances (e.g. devocalisation) or only offering the bespoke option for a particular case (e.g. a biopsy and staging of a mass before excision). Keeping your hands clean maintains the practitioner's integrity and sends a clear message to owners about what the veterinary professional feels is their duty to their animal. But it has the disadvantage of missing opportunities to help the individual patient. So, when we choose such *clean hands* options, we should try to protect the animal's welfare as much as possible, for example by providing analgesia or taking other steps such as reporting the owner to legal authorities.

The alternative option is to "get your hands dirty". One can decide what should be done based on the specific patient's circumstances, even if this choice would not have to be done in a perfect world. This might involve providing a *tactical overtreatment* that you would sooner was never provided (e.g. tail-docking a puppy because we expect that otherwise the owner would do it themselves inhumanely) or providing an imperfect option for a particular case (e.g. excising a mass without a prior biopsy). As another example, we may provide a performance-enhancing neurectomy on a racehorse who will otherwise be sold for meat. Getting your hands dirty maximises the patient's welfare through bespoke practice. But it has the disadvantages that it tacitly endorses the problem and could lead to mistreatment being provided commonly or systematically. So, when we choose such *dirty hands* options, we should offset the welfare harms, for example by lobbying against tail-docking or funding horse rehoming charities, and by informing the owner that they are being imperfect so they may change their future behaviour.

Veterinary professionals can feel uncomfortable providing such tactical overtreatment. However, it is valuable to keep in mind that such options are not mistreatment *for the veterinary professional* because they are the bespoke option for the particular patient in its specific circumstances (e.g. having that owner). The chosen option may be mistreatment *for the owner*, because they are failing to make a welfare-focused decision. The fault lies with the owner, not the veterinary professional. To put it another way, the bespoke treatment is contextually justified by the owner's imperfections.

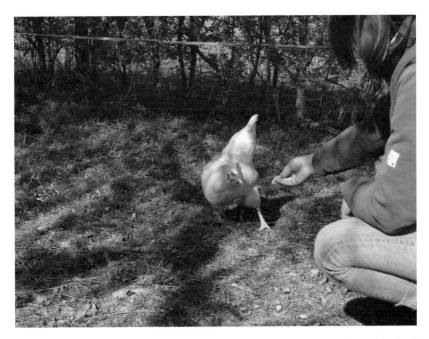

Figure 4.10 An owner may want to show care by hand-feeding chickens, but for fearful chickens, caringness may require more hands-off husbandry. (Courtesy of James Yeates.)

In some cases, clients' wishes coincide with what is best for their animal's welfare (Section 2.5). Where owners are welfare-focused, veterinary professionals can have a collaborative relationship with their clients. One can advise reasonable options and work with owners to decide which of those is best through joint decision-making. Where possible, this approach therefore helps the patient and the client.

Sometimes when owners' expressed wishes do not coincide with what is best for their animal's welfare, joint decision-making can reveal owners' *deeper* wishes which do coincide. Owners may *think* they want one option because they do not know the details, but their deeper wishes would actually favour another option. For example, an owner may ask for a certain medication that the veterinary professional thinks would be mistreatment for a disease. In fact, the owner's deeper wish is for a cure for the disease. Given suitable information that this requires a different therapy, the owner may change their mind and request this treatment instead. Similarly, an owner who is concerned about money may ask for cheaper options. But there may be win-win options that both benefit the animal and save money (e.g. decreasing lameness or mastitis). As another example, a hobby-farmer who wants their chickens to have a good life may think they should show it hands-on love like a pet, but might be persuaded that the chickens may prefer more independence (Figure 4.10). Thus, joint decision-making can help to make clients' and patients' interests coincide.

Another dilemma is when clients' choices do not fit with what the veterinary professional thinks is good for them. For example, some clients may choose to fund very expensive treatments that they seem unable to afford. There is a temptation to overrule their decisions in these cases. However, whatever authority veterinary professionals have regarding animals, we cannot claim to make better decisions than the client concerning the clients themselves. Veterinary professionals should leave the client-focused elements of the decision to the client. If an informed and competent owner wants something that is in the animal's interests, we cannot refuse it because we think another option is better for them. Instead, we must involve the clients in the decision-making in order to represent their own viewpoint.

4.8 Joint Decision-Making

Traditional approaches to decision-making involve both the veterinary professional and the client, but as two separate processes of decision-making (Figure 4.11). There are interactions when each party provides information or influences the other, but they do not share the decision-making process. Specifically, we often think that of ourselves as having privileged wisdom that means our decisions are always *correct*. We then try to implement our decisions paternalistically through communication aimed at *conversion* of the owner to the right decision. The owner's role is to receive, accept and enact our decisions. When they do not, we consider them disobedient or noncompliant.

An alternative approach is to view consultations as meetings between experts, who are jointly involved in the whole process of making an agreed decision. Joint decision-making aims for a more equal clinician–client agreement on welfare issues called *welfare concordance*. Welfare concordance involves more than just agreement about the actual options chosen (which is all that is needed for valid consent). Welfare concordance involves agreement about all of the steps involved in welfare-focused decision-making: it requires shared awareness of the problem, agreed interpretation, concurring evaluations and mutual decision-making processes.

Joint decision-making directly uses owners' knowledge of their animals, constraints, motivations, barriers, complementary ideas about health and welfare and modes of interpretation and evaluation. Joint decision-making can encourage owners to engage with the final decisions, and thus achieve welfare improvements. This may make them more likely to present their animals, fund and consent to treatments, administer medications and monitor for complications and relapses. Joint decisions may therefore have higher quality and effectiveness than unilateral decisions. It can also increase client satisfaction.

Joint decision-making models are not appropriate for every case. In emergency situations, there is no time to have sufficiently complex discussions. Some owners need to be directed or even coerced (e.g. by legal interventions). Other owners may want to leave the decision-making to the veterinary professionals. This applies in

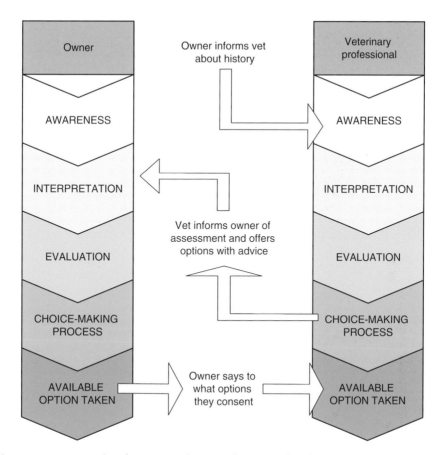

Figure 4.11 Examples of interactions between decision-making by an owner and a veterinary professional.

human medicine as well, where about 50% of intensive care patients' proxies did not want to be involved in decision-making (Azoulay *et al.* 2004). Shared decision-making may work best where there are long-standing and personal client–clinician relationships, as is often the case in veterinary practice.

Joint decision-making is a well-recognised approach in human medicine, and we can learn from human medics' and patients' experiences (see "Selected further reading"). However, human medicine treats the client as having the ultimate authority about their welfare. Veterinary practice is usually primarily concerned with our patients' interests rather than our clients. So our joint decision methods should not be similarly client-focused. This means we should (as with all things) be careful in how we draw upon joint decision-making resources used in human medicine.

Nevertheless, there are some lessons we can learn from human medicine. In particular, human medicine has developed a plethora of *patient decision-aids*. These can be used alongside advice and discussion, and appear to improve decision

---

Box 4.5   Principles for joint decision-aid design.

a. Eliciting information from clients
b. Helping the veterinarian understand the client's point of view
c. Explicitly acknowledging the client's expertise
d. Facilitating personal contact between veterinary professional and client
e. Promoting client's ownership of the problem, process and outcomes
f. Directing the form and content of owners' assessment to key needs
g. Encouraging clients to make written commitments
h. Considering assessment relative to inputs
i. Considering assessment relative to social norms
j. Facilitating discussions of barriers and benefits
k. Facilitating feedback

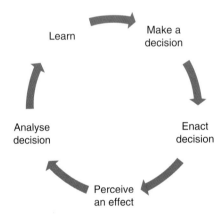

Figure 4.12   A circular model of clients' learning (based on Tate 2003).

quality. These decision-aids can provide facts about the condition, options and outcomes, help to elucidate patients' evaluations of the outcomes and guide patients in the steps of deliberation so that they can make a choice that matches their informed values. Many decision-aids have been catalogued and evaluated by the Cochrane Collaboration, and lots are found on the internet (O'Connor *et al.* 2007). Principles for designing joint decision-aids are given in Box 4.5.

One should not think of joint decision-making as a single event, within a single consultation. Clients will learn from previous experiences, and one can build up relationships and dialogues, gradually increasing their understanding, involvement and mutual trust. One useful model is to consider owners as having a learning circle in which later decisions are based on the results of earlier ones (Figure 4.12). Recognising clients' previous experiences is therefore vital to joint decision-making.

Summary and key recommendations

- There are big deals and there are little matters and the time spent should be proportionate. Sometimes, we can use intuition and emotions to make decisions. However, we may have biases, such as an intervention bias, diagnosis fetishism, unthinkingly copying human medicine and ego-focuses. Structured methods can make us more rational, unbiased and transparent.
- We should offer only reasonable options. Undertreatment is where animals do not get treatments worth having. Overtreatment is where they get treatments worse than no treatment or euthanasia (i.e. if they give an animal a life-worth-avoiding). There are no definitive and comprehensive lists of overtreatment or undertreatment because textbook treatments must be adapted as bespoke practice for each patient, based on future welfare evaluations of each option.
- Decisions affecting multiple patients can be approached by considering each individual, by aggregating intensity, duration, numbers and probability for all animals or by focusing on hierarchical priorities, such as avoiding any animal having a life-worth-avoiding. We should not harm our patients to benefit others, for example through experimental therapies that are not in the patient's interests. We should try to avoid welfare dilemmas and offset any harms to other animals.
- The interests of humans can *constrain* decisions without *construing* them, so they should be side effects. Joint decision-making can help to make better decisions. Practitioners should take full responsibility for their own decisions and cannot legitimately transfer their animal welfare account to their employers, colleagues or owners. Other people can affect bespoke treatment choices, by contextually justifying us getting our hands dirty.

Selected further reading

Our responsibilities are described by Tannenbaum (1993), Rollin (2006a) and Yeates (2009a). Euthanasia is discussed by Rollin (2006b), McMillan (1998) and Yeates (2010c). The life-worth-living concept is discussed in FAWC (2009), Wathes (2010) and Yeates (2011b, 2012b), and death by Yeates (2009b). QALYs in human medicine are discussed by Harris (1987), Edgar *et al.* (1998) and Prieto and Sacristán (2003). Radical surgery is discussed by Lascelles and Main (2002), cosmetic surgery by Morton (1992) and Brown (1998) and kidney transplants by Webster (2005). Decision quality is discussed by Sepucha *et al.* (2004) and joint decision-making and concordance by Coulter (1999), Charles *et al.* (1999) and Weiss and Britten (2003).

Achieving Animal Welfare Goals

5

5.1 Tackling Pathological and Iatrogenic Causes of Feelings

Having determined how to make a good welfare-based decision, it is worth considering what those decisions might be. This chapter considers what actions veterinary professionals can actually do, in order to improve animals' welfare, by maximising the beneficial effects of owners (Sections 5.2, 5.3, 5.4, 5.5, 5.6 and 5.7) and practitioners (Sections 5.8 and 5.9). Most obviously, veterinary professionals can tackle health-related issues. Diseases and injuries can be cured by medical and surgical interventions (Figure 5.1) or prevented by prophylactic treatments such as antiparasitics, vaccination, neutering and breeding health schemes. Euthanasia can reduce and prevent any pathological causes of welfare problems.

Veterinary treatments can also directly affect animals' feelings. There are increasingly good regimes for analgesia, anti-pruritics, anti-emetics and protocols for anti-anxiety drugs such as tricyclics (e.g. clomipramine), serotonin-reuptake-inhibitors (e.g. fluoxetine), monoamine oxidase inhibitors (e.g. selegiline) and benzodiazepines (e.g. alprazolam) and pheromones (e.g. Podberscek *et al.* 1999; King *et al.* 2000, 2004; Crowell-Davis *et al.* 2003; Landsberg *et al.* 2003; Mills *et al.* 2003; Sheppard and Mills 2003; Levine *et al.* 2007). Palliative care is an advancing area of veterinary practice, due to medical advances, owners' increasing willingness-to-pay and trends in human medicine like the Hospice Movement. The use of palliative therapies is now common, and consideration is being given to routine use of other palliative treatments, such as anti-nausea medication for chemotherapy patients or canine vestibular syndrome, the equivalents of which can cause unpleasant feelings of nausea and

Animal Welfare in Veterinary Practice, First Edition. James Yeates.
© 2013 Universities Federation for Animal Welfare. Published 2013 by Blackwell Publishing Ltd.

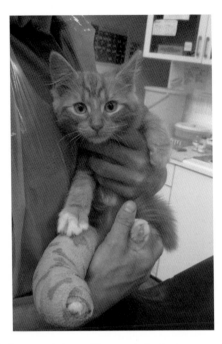

Figure 5.1 Vets can help animals by tackling pathological causes of poor welfare. (Courtesy of RSPCA Bristol.)

unbalance in humans (Farmer & Mustian 1963; Gill *et al.* 2006). Palliative therapy is often thought of as a minor element of veterinary practice (we veterinary professionals like to cure things). But completely effective palliative therapy can be as good as curative therapy from a welfare perspective. Palliative therapy should be routine. Painkillers should be routinely given for all painful conditions, including chronic conditions, visceral pain and pain in farm animals.

There is a danger that palliative therapy perpetuates the lives of suffering animals by inhibiting a euthanasia decision from the owner. Firstly, offering palliative care provides owners with an attractive option which sounds acceptable, even if it does not raise the animal's quality-of-life to the level of a life-worth-living, and which allows owners to defer making an irreversible decision. Palliative care can therefore cause a major iatrogenic harm by perpetuating a life-worth-avoiding. Practitioners need to balance advocating the palliation of suffering and not perpetuating a poor quality life, for example by strongly recommending euthanasia, providing only short-term prescriptions of treatments and being prepared to report owners who refuse consent to authorities.

In contrast, veterinary treatments can also directly affect the *symptoms* of welfare harms. For example, behavioural modification can alter animals' behaviours, without addressing the underlying causes. Such treatments may be in the interests of the client. But they are not in the interests of the animal if they only

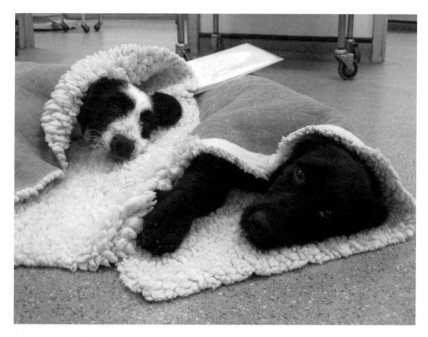

Figure 5.2 Providing good post-operative pain relief is an important part of surgical skill. (Courtesy of RSPCA Bristol.)

alleviate signs, because of the potential for iatrogenic harms. Purely symptomatic treatment is therefore not welfare-focused, except where it addresses behaviours that are the *causes* of harms (e.g. avoiding self-mutilation). For this reason, it might be better to consider this discipline of veterinary medicine not as *behavioural medicine* but as *animal psychiatry*.

Good welfare-focused choices can also improve welfare by reducing iatrogenic harms. Analgesia can often control pain from operations, and surgical descriptions increasingly include laudable recommendations on routine analgesia usage (Figure 5.2). Routine analgesia does not imply one-size-fits-all medication, and recent years have seen a focus on using multimodal, combinatorial regimes and tailored regimes for individual patients.

Practitioners may also take steps to reduce the problems caused by hospitalisation, isolation and stable rest. We should provide sufficient bedding, keep ambient temperatures within patient's thermoneutral zones (and ill animals may be comfortable in different temperature), try to replicate patients' normal routines where possible, and use pleasant ambient aromas, species-specific pheromones or familiar smells (Figure 5.3). Environmental enrichment, including human company (Figure 5.4), can also help reduce stress and even improve health (Table 5.1).

Veterinary professionals can minimise vet-fear by taking care over their comportment and handling. This involves avoiding methods that can cause pain

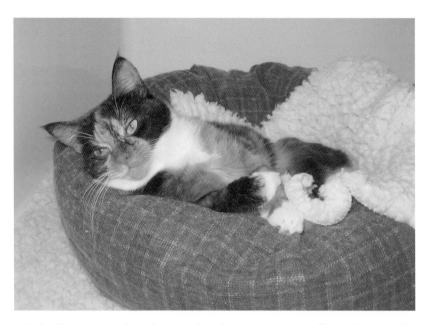

Figure 5.3 Pheromones in kennels may reduce the iatrogenic harm of hospitalisation. (Courtesy of RSPCA Bristol.)

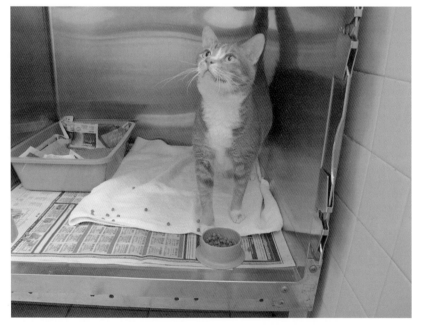

Figure 5.4 Appropriate human contact can provide enrichment for some hospitalised patients. (Courtesy of SPCA Hong Kong.)

Table 5.1 Key inputs that can reduce iatrogenic harms of hospitalisation for dogs.

Input	Feelings produced	Feelings avoided	Selected references
Toys	Mental stimulation Relaxation	Boredom	Hetts *et al.* (1992); Wells (2004); Wells and Hepper (1992), (2000); Hubrecht (1993, 1995); Loveridge (1998); Rooney *et al.* (2009)
Auditory stimulation (e.g. classical music)	Relaxation	Disturbance	Ladd *et al.* (1992); Wells *et al.* (2002)
Olfactory stimulation (e.g. own smell, pheromones, chamomile)	Relaxation	Anxiety	Graham *et al.* (2005)
Visual or olfactory contact with other dogs	Fellow-feeling	Loneliness	Hubrecht (1993); Wells and Hepper (1998)
Human interaction	Amae	Loneliness	Hennessy *et al.* (1998, 2002); Coppola *et al.* (2006); Loveridge (1998)

(e.g. punishment and picking rodents up by their tails) or fear (e.g. intimidating eye contact, unnecessary invasions of body space or flight zones and sudden movements). In some cases, patients should see specific staff where they have a preference or where certain colleagues have previously performed unpleasant interventions. Where possible, vet-fear can be decreased or prevented by longer-term efforts, such as providing pleasant experiences (Simpson 1997), especially during *socialisation periods* (Lindsay 2005). For example, dogs can be trained to be muzzled through pleasant and gradual small steps (Rooney *et al.* 2009), and this may be done by owners at home. Some patients may even end up enjoying coming into the practice (and such *vet-love* is a good success criterion for one's handling skills).

Efforts to minimise iatrogenic harms effectively constitute treatments. So they can cause more iatrogenic harms. Thus, veterinary professionals need not only to consider how to minimise the effects of their treatments for pathological causes of feelings, but also how to minimise the effects of their treatments for iatrogenic causes of feelings (and so on).

5.2 Tackling Owner Causes of Feelings

Owners can assist or frustrate our efforts to address pathological and iatrogenic causes of unpleasant feelings. It is usually the animal's owner who calls a veterinary

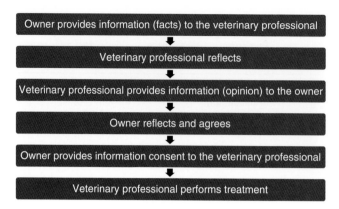

Figure 5.5 Idealised picture of client–clinician communication.

professional out to see the animal or brings it to the surgery, provides a history, consents to the procedures and pays for the treatment. They then administer medication, comply with recommendations and bring the animal in for follow-up checks or if something goes wrong. Owners are even more significant in our efforts to tackle owner-related causes of welfare harms. For these cases, owner changes are the main – or only – way to improve patients' welfare, for example to improve husbandry (e.g. diet or care) or human–animal interactions (e.g. exercise and training). There are a number of different ways the *owner factor* can be managed, including legal, economic and communicative methods.

Legal methods include refusing to give a treatment that only veterinary professionals can legally provide or reporting the owner to authorities for criminal offences. In some cases, one can rehome the animal, so that a new owner has the legal property rights to make decisions about the animal. Indeed, owners are so important that sometimes the best way to improve an animal's welfare is to get the animal *another* owner.

Economic methods include charging for overtreatment, providing subsidised or free treatment, utilising charities money and using conventional commercial marketing techniques that *hard sell* animal welfare goals.

Communicative methods involve utilising the interactions within the consultation. Communication is an important element of veterinary work, and evidence from human medicine suggests better communication is associated with fewer errors, higher patient satisfaction, greater compliance and less litigation (DiMatteo *et al.* 1993; Stewart 1995; Silverman *et al.* 2005).

We tend to imagine communication to be a rational, cognitive exercise, where the owner provides information, upon which we reflect, and then we provide information and authoritative opinion, upon which the owner reflects and then agrees (Figure 5.5). But this is a myth. Communication is a matter of myriad

---

Box 5.1 Elements of social marketing strategies.

P	Use of *prompts* to remind clients
I	Active *involvement* of the person in the decision
N	Use of *norms*, i.e. relative to what other people do, or other animals
O	Gaining *ownership* in the process and outcomes
C	Use of *credible community leaders* and personal *contact*
C	Getting *commitment*, ideally in writing
H	*Hooks* to draw the client into the discussion and decision-making
I	*Identifying* the people most likely to change
O	Displaying *owner benefits* and addressing *owner barriers*

---

cultural and psychological factors (Fielding 1995), and involves a range of sophisticated personal skills that require intuition and emotional intelligence. Veterinary professionals used to have to learn such skills as they went along (Adams & Frankel 2007), but veterinary communication is developing as a field of research and education. This education is often informed by human medicine, although veterinary communication is different, since it involves discussion about a third party. Communication in small animal work is more similar to paediatrics, although non-human animals are different to children.

One area of communication research that is especially relevant to achieving animal welfare goals is *social marketing*. This field concerns what strategies can best change how people *behave* (it was largely developed through efforts in environmental and health fields such as recycling and anti-smoking campaigns). Because social marketing is concerned with motivating behaviour change, it could be especially useful in helping us work out how to achieve owner behaviour changes that can improve their animals' welfare. Many different communication tactics have been suggested for social marketing campaigns (Box 5.1).

Using these methods, veterinary professionals can guide and assist owners through their decision-making process. But before considering how veterinary professionals can best communicate with clients, it is worth remembering that good vet–client communication also requires owners to communicate well. In 2004, the Association of the British Pharmaceutical Industry produced a list of points relating to how patients should communicate. An expanded and adapted form for veterinary professionals is given in Box 5.2. Unfortunately, and evidently, most clients receive no communication skills training. They too have to learn as they go along. Fortunately, we can help them to learn by advising them on their communication. At the very least, we can encourage them to be honest and candid. Of course, this communication-about-communication needs especially good communication skills.

Box 5.2   Client virtues.

Clients should:

- Come prepared
- Be punctual and presentable
- Control their animal and children
- Be honest
- Be realistic about their limitations (e.g. finances and animal handling ability)
- Respect veterinary practice staff, other clients and animals
- Listen carefully
- Make efforts to remember (e.g. taking notes)
- Speak enough – but not too much
- Give relevant information
- Avoid giving irrelevant information
- Make only reasonable demands
- Ask questions
- Take advice
- Accept bespoke solutions where they represent compromises due to owner limitations (e.g. finances)
- Raise any concerns or queries
- Be prepared to finance reasonable treatment options
- Pay bills promptly

5.3 Improving Owners' Assessments

Veterinary professionals can guide owners' assessment for all three of the steps involved. We can increase owners' awareness by informing owners about the existence of welfare problems. We can improve their interpretation by explaining what symptoms mean in terms of animal welfare, providing diagnoses and aetiologies, describing prognoses, treatment options and possible sequelae, and explaining the implications of options in terms of their costs and effect on owners' lifestyle. We can also provide useful background knowledge to improve their prior understanding, guidance on their interpretation and specific advice to target any emotional biases. Giving information to owners is an important method for changing owners' behaviour (Patronek *et al.* 1996) and reducing non-compliance (e.g. Stimson 1974).

There are several limitations to providing information to owners. One is their comprehension, which may depend on their general knowledge, linguistic abilities, prior understanding and any emotional biases. To address these, veterinary professionals should provide information in ways owners can understand. What information we provide should focus on what information owners want and need to know in order to make the best decision (e.g. information on prices, prognoses and welfare implications), and not on unimportant information (e.g. the exact nature of the procedure, the names of the drugs or the exact diagnosis).

Owners often struggle to understand scientific data that may underlie veterinary professionals' interpretations. But they can appreciate how they would feel if they were in a similar situation to their animal. This can make critical anthropomorphism a valuable *communication* tool (regardless of its usefulness as a welfare assessment method). As discussed in Chapters 1 and 3, this approach should be used with caution, because excessive anthropomorphism can lead to inappropriate treatment decisions.

Owners also frequently struggle to understand probabilities, especially very large or small risks, or where the outcomes that may occur are emotionally charged. It can be useful to express a risk in terms of how often the relevant outcome would be expected to occur (e.g. 1 animal in 10 is alive after 6 months). Where owners are disproportionately concerned about one risk and not another, it can be useful to compare the *relative risks* between one treatment option and another or between a benefit and a harm. For example, a radical surgery may have a 1% chance of extending life but a 100% chance of causing significant pain and frustration.

Other limitations of communicating information concern the veterinary professionals ourselves. We may fail to devote enough time to giving, explaining or repeating information. We may use terms that make owners less receptive, defensive or scared. Indeed, even the term *welfare* can seem like an accusatory term, especially in those countries with well-known welfare laws. We may spend too long explaining irrelevant details (which we find interesting) or use unnecessarily technical language or acronyms. In fact, these technical terms can be confusing even if we also use commonplace words alongside, and it is often better to use only the lay word.

One can raise owners' awareness through explicit joint welfare assessment. Screening methods allow veterinary professionals to demonstrate the broad scope of issues that may affect an animal's welfare and to give advice even where there is no immediate reason to do so without seeming interfering or hard selling. Welfare assessment by owners may encourage them to seek veterinary treatment. Such engagement appears to work in human medicine (Roter 2000; King & Moulton 2006; Griffiths *et al.* 2007), including human paediatrics (Janicke *et al.* 2001), and in farm animal welfare initiatives (Catley *et al.* 2002; Vaarst *et al.* 2007).

A participatory tool was recently developed for dog welfare assessment in practice (Figure 5.6), and the designer found it very useful both in raising issues efficiently and in getting clients to commit to changing how they care for their animal (Yeates *et al.* 2011), as shown in Figure 5.7. Other veterinary professionals also found the tool useful, but less so. This suggests that it is useful to design one's own tool for one's own clients. By the same logic that we have said applies to owners, being involved and engaged in designing a tool means you can tailor it to your own style and clients, and have *ownership* of the tool. It is good to design, or adapt, your own welfare assessment tool for use in your own practice.

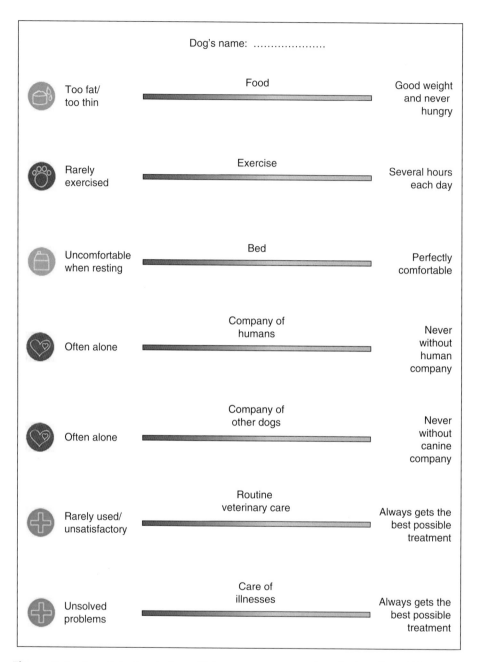

Figure 5.6 A *participatory tool* on which owners can assess their dog's welfare. (After Yeates *et al.* 2011.)

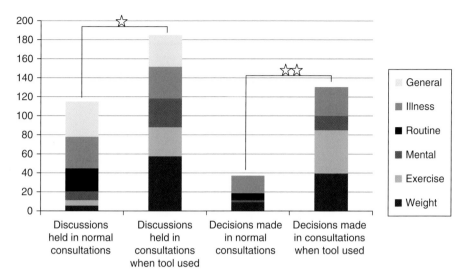

Figure 5.7 Number of discussions owners had with their veterinary professional and decisions they made (per 100 consultations) during normal consultations and during consultations using the participatory tool. (After Yeates *et al.* 2011.)

Other participatory methods could be adapted from methods used in rural communities and developing countries. For example, owners could be asked to rate how good their animal's welfare is based on six outcome measures, using the *welfare circle* in Figure 5.8. More pictorial owners might be asked to draw a map of their animal's environment, or the animal's body, highlighting any actual and potential problems. More mathematical owners could draw a graph of their animal's welfare over time (e.g. during a chronic illness), including any significant events that have changed it.

5.4 Improving Owners' Evaluations and Choices

Veterinary professionals can also help owners to evaluate and make welfare-focused choices. Recognising owners' benefits and barriers allows you to correct erroneous assumptions and point out benefits they may have missed. It can be useful to highlight pros and cons, and one can create decision-making aids that list benefits and risks, using either pre-prepared tools or bespoke methods.

Social marketing research suggests that we are all motivated by other people, either consciously or subconsciously. Given the social expectation about animal welfare, owners may wish to avoid criticism for failing to look after their animal. Veterinary professionals can utilise this motivation to enhance welfare contagion, by reminding owners of the societal morals, by bringing farmers together to discuss welfare issues and by providing feedback that rank farms' welfare scores.

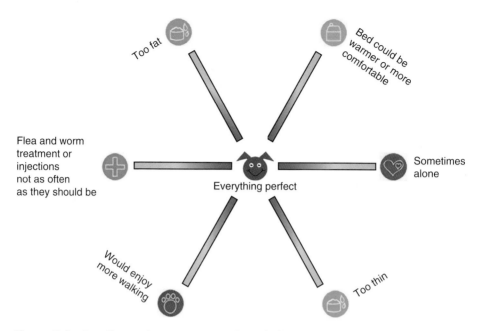

Figure 5.8 A *welfare circle* participatory tool on which owners can assess their dog's welfare.

Veterinary professionals can also spread contagion to our clients by using our position as *key opinion leaders* based on our recognised expertise, our role in the community, our professional status and our acknowledged responsibilities to put animals' interests before our own. We can also provide advice and act as role models (and veterinary practitioners can set a bad role model, e.g. through inappropriate animal handling).

We should also think it acceptable to hard sell welfare improvements. We should offer the best and not only advocate it but should also use our influence and authority to push the client towards whatever is best for welfare. There are many ways to influence owners, based on the ideas discussed in this chapter (Table 5.2). The idea of *hard selling* may seem distasteful, but if animal welfare is veterinary professionals' primary responsibility, then we should strive to achieve it.

Veterinary professionals' influence also comes from our relationship with the client. Relationships are an important part of health care (Beach & Inui 2006) and improving relations can increase adherence (Brown & Silverman 1999). Making oneself more relationship-oriented requires the use of specific strategies and the development of certain habits (Frankel *et al.* 2003). For example, the strategies in Box 5.3 appear to increase human–patient satisfaction scores (Stein *et al.* 2005) and are applicable to veterinary medicine (Adams & Frankel 2007). This can be more difficult with certain clients, or when communication is through a translator, but not impossible.

Table 5.2 Significant forms of veterinary influence over owners.

Form of influence	Examples
Prominence	Encouraging owners to identify welfare issues
History and education	Choosing specific elements to assess
Memory	Prompts
Presentation of information	Presentation of elements
Moral priming	Choosing specific elements to assess
Human–animal relationship	Highlighting animal's interests
Societal influence	Using social norms
Value-loading information	Choice of terms
Emotional priming	Displaying owner benefits
Engaging in reasoning	Joint decision-making methods
Personal suggestions	Using authority
Encouraging certain opinions	Promoting ownership of the problem
Peer pressure	Personal contact
Coercion	Active involvement
Forcing options	Getting commitment
Owner-based barriers/capacities	Addressing barriers

Box 5.3 The four habits (after Frankel and Stein 1993).

Habit 1: Invest in the beginning
Habit 2: Elicit the owner's/client's perspective
Habit 3: Demonstrate empathy
Habit 4: Invest in the end

Sometimes it is necessary to encourage owners to care more. This can alter their evaluation or their decision-making, for example by making them less concerned about their own interests, more likely to engage with the issue and more determined to achieve the required behavioural changes. This may explain why we use different communication styles for problem-focused versus routine appointments (Shaw et al. 2006). Evidence from human medicine suggests that discussions of empathy can make owners more likely to achieve treatment goals. However, too much concern can lead to *decreased* likelihood, for example where owners are overemotional and cannot make a decision or act (Figure 5.9). So increasing owners' concern should be balanced with not making them too concerned to make good decisions (Tate 2003).

Nevertheless, veterinary professionals can use direct personal appeals. Emotional discussions appear uncommon for both doctors (Myerscough & Ford 1996) and veterinary professionals (Shaw et al. 2004). But emotions are an important part of

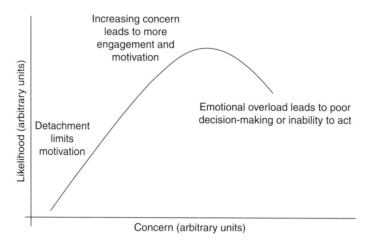

Figure 5.9 Representation of a theoretical relationship between level of owner concern and likelihood to make a decision or a lifestyle change.

medical relationships, and we should listen for evidence of client's emotions and respond to them. Such personal involvement may make us seem more friendly and compassionate, allow us to use our empathy and emotional responses explicitly, help us to discuss clients' emotions more openly and constructively and allow us to consider how their emotions provide benefits and barriers to behaviour changes. One concept used in human medicine, but not employed in veterinary practice is that of *narrative medicine*. This can be characterised as "medicine practised with the narrative competence to recognise, absorb, interpret, and be moved by the stories of illness" (Charon 2006). The narrative approach can support and augment caring relationships, because they involve the client being empathetic and non-objective: indeed some argue that they require the clinician to be willing to suffer. Even if one does not go that far, exploring the broader life setting of the client and pet allows a veterinarian to gain a greater understanding of the pet's illness (McMillan 2002).

5.5 Improving Owners' Achievements

Owners may accept recommendations but fail to make the required behaviour changes. This failure may concern not giving a medicine, not returning for revisits or post-operative checks or failing to make a lifestyle change such as decreasing food or increasing exercise. Fortunately, a lot of work has gone into finding ways to improve compliance within both human and veterinary medical fields.

It is valuable to make owners' aims coincide with their animals' interests. Highlighting benefits can help owners to sustain their motivation by keeping these advantages in mind. Highlighting likely barriers can prepare owners so that they are not surprised or daunted when they encounter them and feel empowered to successfully tackle them. Some owners may be overwhelmed if faced by very complicated protocols or demanding lifestyle changes. It can be better to break these down into feasible *small steps*. For example, one can separate the administration of insulin injections into smaller steps of drawing-up, tenting skin, injecting (e.g. using sterile water at first), recognising symptoms of hypoglycaemia and hyperglycaemia, timing, etc. Similarly, one can suggest less ambitious dieting or exercise regimes and gradually build them up.

Achievement may also be increased by helping owners to remember the decisions after the consultation. It is good practice to summarise and reiterate three key points at the end of the consultation. One can also set up prompts and reminders to give feedback on improvements (Seligman & Darley 1977), for example by linking the drug administration to a daily (a news programme) or monthly event (the first of each month). Alternatively, you can set up a system to telephone, text or email the client with reminders, although such practice efforts must be sustainable and realistic.

There is also benefit in continuing the relationship beyond each consultation. One can check that things are going well (and screen for welfare problems), and provide feedback on owners' achievements, which can also lead to increased behaviour change (Seligman & Darley 1977). These methods may increase compliance with the recommendations given.

Even more important than compliance is concordance. Owners cannot be expected to simply implement *our* decisions. They have to make their *own* decisions and formulate a genuine intention that they will actually fulfil. This requires that they are involved and engaged with the decision-making process and recognise it as their own, so that they personally endorse and identify with the decision and take personal moral responsibility for the problems, the process of its resolution and the final outcomes. This requires joint decision-making with realistic aims as to what quality of decision can be attained. Owners may have many barriers and biases to making welfare-focused decisions, and combating all of these may require being less ambitious not only about what the owner might be expected to do, but also what they might be expected to think and to decide. This makes it especially useful to take owners through the process gradually, because just as owners may be more able to take *small steps* in their lifestyle changes, so may they may be more able to make small steps in changing how they make decisions. It may be easier to reach concordance about basic *reasoning building blocks*, such as what is important for animals or how a sign should be interpreted, and then to build up into decisions.

Concordance may also be improved by reminding owners of their reasoning. Our *three key points* tend to relate to the final decision (e.g. rest, remedy, revisit), but we can help owners to remember why they made those decisions by reminding them not only of the treatment plan but also of the ways to observe welfare problems, background information and the reasoning that underlay the decision to choose that plan. If an owner later revisits their decision, then they can recall their

---

Box 5.4   Binary criteria for euthanasia of an animal.

[NB: threshold is if any of these are true.]

If the animal:
- Is unable to stand on more than 2+ attempts
- Is inappetent or not drinking for 2+ days
- Is unable to defecate for over 2+ days or urinate for over 24 hours
- Continues to make pain-related vocalisations despite every available analgesia protocol
- Is unwilling to exercise more than 3+ days in a row
- Does not interact with a conspecific (if gregarious species) for 14+ days
- Is in severe pain or distress for 3+ days
- Is cyanotic or markedly dyspnoeic for 1+ hour
- Has a coughing fit 3+ times per waking hour for 3+ days
- Is pyrexic for 4+ days
- Has 1+ seizure every 2+ months

or
- Has no obvious pleasure in its life for 5+ days

and
- It is not possible to otherwise resolve the cause for any of the above

---

working as well as their *conclusions*. This may make them more likely to adhere to the treatment plan, since people may be more likely to agree with a decision if they understand the basis for the decision (Hastie & Dawes 1988). Putting information in writing can decrease one's reliance on owners' memory. Pre-prepared handouts can record pre-decided unilateral choices; joint decisions need to be recorded by bespoke documents co-written by the clinician and owner.

Getting owners to *commit* to their decision requires them to actively and explicitly express an intention. Ideally, this should look at both *now and forever*: owners should say exactly what they are ultimately aiming to achieve and exactly what they will do as a first step. Owners can commit verbally (the ultimate commitment being an explicit promise), although putting commitment in writing appears to increase its potency (Pardini & Katzev 1983–1984). In some cases, it is useful to get owners to commit to a decision *before* that decision has to be made. For example, one can formulate objective criteria for euthanasia such as those in Box 5.4. These criteria may be arbitrary and retrospective, but they can provide an objective way to make owners more likely to give consent at a later time.

5.6 Money Solutions

Economic strategies can alter owners' behaviours, especially by removing financial barriers or highlighting economic benefits.

Veterinary professionals can often get owners to make behavioural changes or fund treatments by identifying *win-win* options that will both improve animal welfare and increase owner profit. However, there can still be two problems. The first is in *demonstrating* that it is a win-win situation. Sometimes, this can involve quite detailed financial discussions, often trying to overcome other barriers an owner may have. The second is in addressing cash-flow issues. Sometimes, owners may be fully aware of the benefits of an investment, but be unable to fund that investment in the short term. Some countries have support groups that can help, otherwise veterinary professionals can sometimes offer to delay invoicing.

Owners' financial limitations can be pre-emptively removed, for example by encouraging owners to get insurance for their animals. The profession needs to work harder to encourage this and to find ways to influence what policies exist and how they are chosen. Veterinary professionals can also address financial barriers by limiting, or reducing, their prices. Practices have to charge, in order to cover costs and a reasonable mark-up. But this mark-up should not prioritise profit over uptake. Prices should be *reasonable*, and not exploit owners' ignorance about veterinary practice and inability to make rational consumer choices. Pricing methods should also avoid misleading clients through tactics like loss leader strategies or dishonestly giving the impression of being budget practices when really being equally or more expensive than competitors.

The ultimate way to avoid financial barriers is to provide subsidised or free treatment for those clients who cannot afford treatment. It may seem unfair that some clients should get cheaper treatment, so a better way to think of this is to provide treatment for certain *patients* (who happen to have owners who will not fund normally priced treatment). Many veterinary professionals find it personally rewarding to spend time or money helping some patients and clients. On a practice level, such pro bono work can also be important for employee health and well-being, since the stress of being unable to treat animals can significantly worsen job satisfaction, and thus employee motivation and retention.

Pro bono work can be cheap (Figure 5.10). It can easily use up practice resources. Consequently, it needs to be limited to certain cases (e.g. emergency treatment or euthanasia) or to a certain cost (e.g. one could set up a limited monthly account for practice pro bono work). Alternatively, pro bono work might be funded by a specific in-house charity, which can be supported by practice fund-raising events or contributions from other clients. Indeed, practices could go further and transparently charge all clients a small surcharge (say 0.1%) which goes to this charity fund – this may even be a win-win for the practice if it makes them seem a more ethical company.

Where neither win-win nor pro bono treatment options are possible, another solution is to offer a range of options to cater for a range of budgets. This is common in many industries; for example, you can purchase a range of quality foodstuffs from *gourmet* through to *economy* products. Similarly, practices may try to give *budget* options. This flexibility can reduce undertreatment by meaning that animals are not left completely untreated. For example, if a farmer whose cow

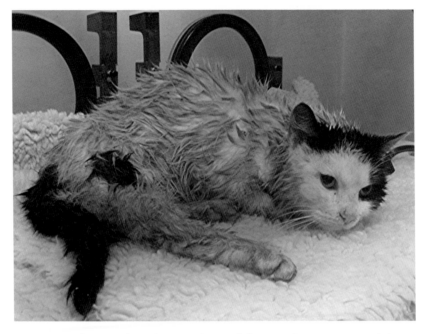

Figure 5.10 Pro bono work can be rewarding and cheap, such as warming and cleaning this hypothermic cat. (Courtesy of RSPCA Bristol.)

has a solar ulcer cannot (or will not) fund expensive treatment, the veterinary professionals can offer claw amputation (rather than nothing). If a horse's owner will not fund colic surgery, the veterinary professionals might offer short-term analgesia or immediate euthanasia. On a wider scale, some practices market themselves as *budget* practices with lower fees and focus on more economical treatments, in order to cater for less affluent owners.

Conversely, avoiding extreme undertreatment by offering cheaper options should not lead to undertreatment because owners use those options when they would otherwise have chosen the better option. So we should make sure we do also offer, and advocate, the best options (Main 2006). One approach is to offer the best option first, and to offer the next best only if that is rejected (Rollin 2006a). The problem with this is that it misses the opportunity of involving the owner in the decision-making because each time it only offers them one choice, which they can only affirm or reject. Thus, this method will not work in cases where the decision-making would benefit from the client's active involvement.

In order to involve the owner meaningfully, it may be necessary to give some indication of *value for money*. This is especially important for the owner *and the animal* where resources are limited, for example where owners have a set budget or a capped insurance policy. In such cases, spending money on, say, an unnecessary out-of-hours call or pre-operative blood test may mean there is no money for later treatment. Thus, even if the earlier options are not overtreatment per se, they lead to undertreatment later on. In welfare terms, value for money can be conceptualised in terms of quality-adjusted-life-periods/dollar, but it is easier to communicate with owners in more qualitative terms, for example by highlighting where treatment is *essential* and *reasonable*.

5.7 Legal Solutions

In some cases, working with the owner through communicative and economic methods are not enough. Some owners are resistant to all information, advice and influence. In these cases, we need to work *against* the owner, by limiting the options they have available. Most obviously, if an owner has broken the law, veterinary professionals can report them to the police or other authority. When an owner is part of a regulated activity (e.g. horseracing or pedigree dog breeding), veterinary professionals also can inform the regulatory body if the owner breaks the activity's rules (e.g. through *doping* or prohibited surgery).

The advantages of reporting an owner are that it can prevent future welfare harms, especially when prosecution leads to the owner losing that animal, being disqualified from keeping any animals, or losing a licence to use animals in certain ways. This advantage may be especially marked when the owner's previous abuse has caused harm to many animals or suffering of considerable intensity, frequency or duration (Figure 5.11). The disadvantages of reporting an owner are twofold. Firstly, reporting an owner risks harming the practice by taking up valuable time in writing reports and court appearances, and possibly by damaging the practice's public relations. Secondly, reporting owners to authorities could risk owners being less likely to seek veterinary attention. Veterinary professionals need to decide whether the advantages outweigh the risks.

One can approach this decision in the same way as other welfare-based decisions. For example, one could estimate the severity and numbers of animals that would be affected by reporting and not reporting. Often, the danger to the practice and future animals is negligible, especially when reports can be genuinely anonymous. In some cases, one might feel it is also important to consider whether the owner caused the welfare harms *deliberately* or *cruelly*. This is important where the law takes it into account, and may also affect how successful other methods of persuasion might be. However, in purely welfare terms, the morality of the owner is irrelevant, and in some cases it is unfortunately necessary to prosecute people who are simply unaware, overemotional or misguided.

A subtler method of influencing the client is to inform them that their behaviour would constitute a criminal offence. This information can help to motivate the client, both because the law is an indicator of what society considers morally acceptable and because avoiding prosecution is a significant benefit that would coincide with improving their animal's welfare. Depending on the client, you can either present this warning as a helpful piece of advice (that someone else may report them) or as a specific threat (that you will). Plus, of course one can then back it up with actually reporting them.

A different way to restrict an owner's ability to choose an undesirable option is simply to refuse to do it. To put it another way, one should not offer or perform overtreatment on request any more than one should offer mistreatment. For procedures that are legally restricted to veterinary professionals, veterinary refusals

(a)   (b)

(c)

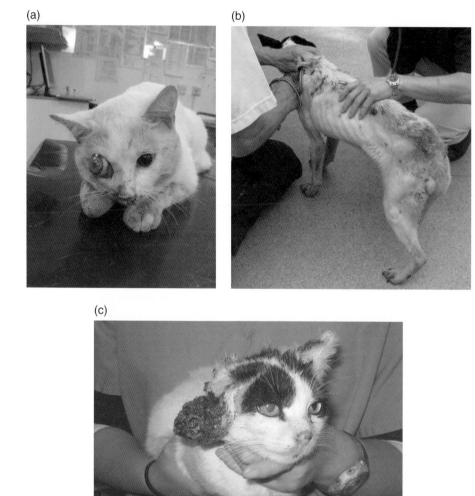

Figure 5.11 Some cruelty cases have caused suffering of considerable (a) intensity, (b) frequency or (c) duration, such as repeated flare-ups on multiple body-parts. (Courtesy of RSPCA Bristol.)

mean the owner cannot provide the treatment legally, and therefore hopefully chooses a better option that is offered. However, this tactic is ineffective when the owner can obtain the treatment from another veterinary professional, and potentially bad for the animal if that other veterinary professional is less welfare-focused (indeed this may be why they are providing the treatment). It is better for these situations to be prevented by our interactions with other veterinary professionals.

5.8 Colleagues

Achieving animal welfare can often depend on cooperation between the practice team (Figure 5.12). It can also depend on how other veterinary professionals make their decisions, and what advice and options they offer to clients. Effective communication and cooperation with colleagues can overcome practices' barriers to promoting welfare. As with owners, this can involve working with, on and against one's colleagues using communicative, economic and legal means.

When a veterinary professional wishes to influence a colleague's decisions, one has several options. One is to do nothing. This is easy but ineffective. Another option is direct communication such as writing treatment plans with thresholds for decisions (e.g. recoding a plan that euthanasia will be considered if a downer cow or cast horse is still not up within 8 hours). In most cases, communication should be done tactfully and ideally proactively before cases happen, rather than criticising past events. In more

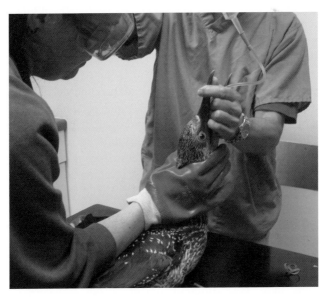

Figure 5.12 Practice teamwork requires cooperation between colleagues. (Courtesy of RSPCA Bristol.)

extreme cases, clinicians can whistle-blow to a practice boss, the police, the veterinary regulatory body, or the public media. Such whistle-blowing can be very harmful to both the accused and the accuser, through retribution or even job-loss, so it should be a last resort for serious issues that cannot be safely discussed in other ways (Yeates 2012c).

Communication can also help to discuss current practices. Outdated or erroneous practices may become established and entrenched (especially if some alternatives have been unsuccessfully tried). Other such practices may be propagated by practice culture, role models, employers and imperfect standard operative procedures. Sometimes it takes an outsider or new member of staff to see the possibilities, although their insights should be balanced with the knowledge of established staff about the circumstances of the practice and its clients. Mutual education can help all colleagues to feel competent in giving advice on welfare issues. As well as discussing clinical cases in medical terms, we can share animal welfare knowledge and discuss interpretations, evaluations, clinical options and communication. If necessary, such topics can be formally included in case discussions, with an agenda to include iatrogenic harms, such as pain and hospitalisation, and factors that affect achieving welfare goals, such as owner barriers and communication methods.

Coordination between colleagues can prevent veterinary professionals performing a given intervention because they fear a colleague may otherwise do so. Coordination can also help increase efficiency and thus save time, for example through standard operating procedures (SOPs). SOPs should not mandate the overtreatment of any cases or systematic undertreatment (and treatment SOPs should never be implemented to increase revenue). They need to allow clinicians to have the flexibility to make good decisions and to achieve joint decisions. One useful approach is to say they are the *default plan*, deviations from which should be justified by reference to the particular case. SOPs can also be used to coordinate communication methods, consultation styles or welfare assessment protocols.

As well as recognising the barriers, it is also useful to recognise the benefits that colleagues might obtain from achieving welfare goals. Some welfare improvements are win-win solutions that benefit patients, practice and personnel, such as proactively marketing products or services like flea-control, worming, dental hygiene, microchipping and neutering. Practices can also use economic methods to increase these benefits, for example through incentive schemes such as performance-related pay, that tie welfare goals to employees' personal remuneration. These incentives are usually linked to turn-over or profit, such as profit-related pay, but they could be linked to other welfare goals. Such schemes are only acceptable if they are done to improve welfare (with personal benefits as a side effect), so practices must avoid incentivising overtreatment.

Collaboration can help practices to achieve more ambitious and proactive welfare goals. Colleagues may feel that there is some salient issue that merits attention from all staff, such as promoting vaccination, puppy classes, weight clinics or geriatric checks. Everyone may have different priorities, but practices can be formal prioritisation methods, as described in Section 6.5, or more participatory methods like those described in Section 5.3. For example, everyone can collaborate as a group to draw cherries on a tree (Figure 5.13) with big cherries representing actions

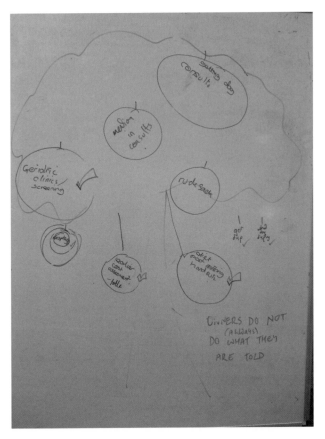

Figure 5.13 Staff at an anonymous practice identified easy and effective actions by pictorially representing them. (Courtesy of RSPCA Bristol.)

that will have a big effect and low-hanging fruits denoting easier actions. The practice can then prioritise those actions that will be easiest and/or most effective.

Practices can then measure the effectiveness of their programme through *clinical governance* based on welfare audit. Human quality-of-life assessment is now a part of a clinical audit in human clinical governance (Sanders *et al.* 1998). Clinical governance may be especially important for developing practitioners. But it is also important for more established practitioners. The learning circle can mean that experience may make us become set in our ways and inflexible. The link between self-esteem and risk-aversion described in Chapter 2 may make more eminent veterinary professionals insufficiently cautious about iatrogenic harms.

Screening audits can identify complications such as anaesthetic reactions. Gauging audits can help to assess overall standards. Decision quality audits can measure how often clients arrive at informed choices, using indicators such as the consistency in take-up of options between the patients of different clinicians (Wennberg 2002). Variation between practitioners provides a reason to reassess our

> **Box 5.5   Five questions concerning what information is worth obtaining for clinical audit.**
>
> 1. What is important for the animals?
> 2. What information is available to us?
> 3. What available information will help us to make decisions?
> 4. What inefficiencies might the assessment methods cause?
> 5. Is the information measurable over time?

joint decision-making methods. Other audits can evaluate how good we are at making owners change their behaviours, using measures such as client compliance, commitment or product sales. It is important that we select suitable issues to assess and suitable measures with which to assess them, avoiding our biases wherever possible. Parameters should be identifiable, measurable, feasible and relevant (Box 5.5).

5.9 Working on Oneself

Previous sections have discussed how to improve our assessment and choice-making steps. It is also worth considering how to make sure we fulfil our welfare-focused decisions. Like clients and colleagues, we are subject to similar motivations and can achieve our animal welfare goals better if we reflect upon our barriers, benefits, biases and other pressures, and adjust our plans to take these into account. For example, reflection even on seemingly-large barriers can allow them to be circumnavigated (Figures 5.14, 5.15, 5.16 and 5.17).

Communication can also help us to achieve our welfare goals – and to avoid preventing others from achieving theirs. Communication may be especially valuable if we talk to people with differing viewpoints. This may reduce the effect of biases due to our non-representative personal experiences and help us to remain aware of more representative social norms. For example, specialists who have frequent exposure to more radical interventions may benefit from discussion with first-opinion veterinary professionals, paraprofessionals and laypeople.

We can also increase our motivation where it is lacking or subject to excessive pressure from clients or colleagues. One can identify or create benefits, such as rewarding oneself personally for one's achievements or reflecting positively on good outcomes or good deeds. One can minimise vet-focused motivations by dissociating our interests from them. For example, one may give one's profit-related-pay to charity, so that it does not influence one's decision-making. One can minimise one's own forgetfulness by reminding oneself of the decisions, for example by setting up prompts and aide memoirs.

Resisting client pressures can be helped by being confident in your decision-making process and reminding yourself of the underlying logic, for example by

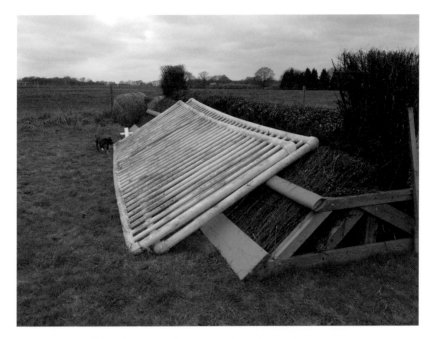

Figure 5.14 We all face barriers. (Courtesy of James Yeates.)

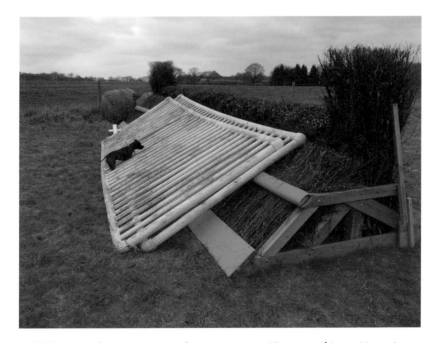

Figure 5.15 Some barriers seem too big to overcome. (Courtesy of James Yeates.)

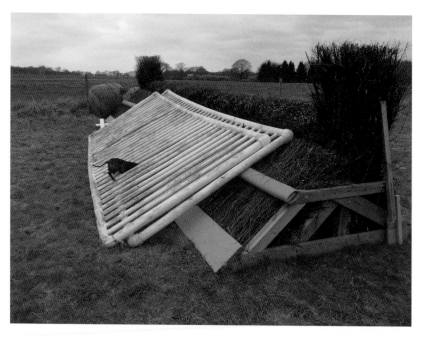

Figure 5.16   Sometimes we can get lost in the immediate difficulties. (Courtesy of James Yeates.)

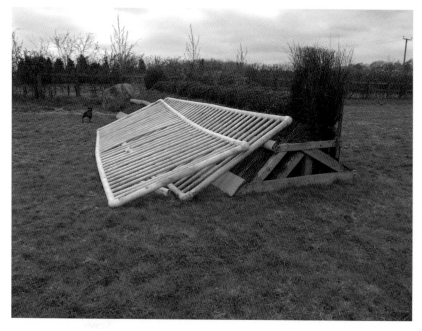

Figure 5.17   But we can often get around many obstacles. (Courtesy of James Yeates.)

formalising one's decision-making and recording it in writing. One can use the law by refusing to provide treatments that could be illegal or contrary to animal welfare. Clinicians who are pressured by owners to perform an illegal intervention can offer to provide that intervention only on the condition the client signs a contract to promise to pay you a veterinary wage for the rest of your life if your transgression leads to you losing your licence to practise.

A commonly perceived barrier for veterinary professionals is staff time. In fact, many practitioners try to find small-talk to establish and build relationships – hence, routine consultations like vaccinations often take almost as long as consultations that discuss a particular problem (Shaw *et al.* 2008) – so we could use this time to ask welfare-based questions that are both directly informative and relationship-building. But, even with this time, we are often rushed and overly busy and feel unable to take on too much extra work. Minimising this barrier requires either identifying win-win options (for practice and animal) or prioritising the most important changes. Limitations in time and resources can be addressed by identifying the most important priorities, in terms of welfare gains and feasibility. We may focus on the most severe cases, i.e. those with the greatest potential welfare improvements. We should also focus on how likely we are to achieve that improvement. It is easy to spend a lot of time on a few cases and on more demanding clients. But we can maximise our welfare achievements by focusing on more achievable welfare improvements – the *low-hanging fruits*.

As one example, it is useful to focus on those owners who are most likely to change their behaviours (McKenzie-Mohr & Smith 1999). This is not to say that one ignores the other clients completely. Effective communication methods are needed for all clients and one should not ignore the worst cases simply because they involve the owners who are least likely to change. But maximising our animal welfare account requires us to maximise our *welfare efficiency*.

How one identifies which clients are most likely to change their behaviour depends on what behaviour one is trying to change. Farmers that appear more successful or modern may be more likely to invest in on-farm improvements. Obese owners may be less likely to successfully control the diet of their animals (unless you can use an owner's obesity to highlight a benefit of exercising their dog more). But in most cases, the most willing-to-change clients are not so easily identified, and one should avoid making over-assumptions. For example, a gushing owner who claims they would "spend whatever is needed" is not always the one most ready to handover the cash later. In the absence of scientific data on how to identify willing clients, this remains part of the art of veterinary practice.

One concept that may help is the Health Belief Model. This is used in human medicine to classify people in terms of how likely they are to take action to improve their own health and was developed to tackle diseases such as TB and HIV (Rosenstock 1974). The model suggests that for change to occur, the patient (in our case, the client) needs to (a) believe the health problem is avoidable, (b) expect that the change in behaviour will avoid the problem and (c) believe that they can change their behaviour in the way required. These depend on six things, summarised in Box 5.6. So

---

Box 5.6   Factors affecting likelihood to change behaviours. (After
Hochbaum 1958; Rosenstock *et al.* 1988; Glanz *et al.* 1997.)

Perceived susceptibility: whether the patient perceives that they are susceptible to the
condition
Perceived severity: how severe the patient perceives the condition to be
Perceived benefits: what benefits the patient perceives there are to changing their behaviour
Perceived barriers: what barriers the patient perceives there are to changing their behaviour
Confidence in self-efficacy: whether the patient is confident in the effectiveness of their
behaviour change
Presence of cues to action: and whether there are sufficient cues to help them
remember the behaviour change

---

when a client is dismissive of the problem, is overly pessimistic about success, seems
completely resigned to the problem or remains resistant to change, one can consider
them less likely to change their behaviour – and focus on other clients.

It is important to reflect on one's previous decisions, while remembering that a
decision may have been correct even if one then suffers *bad welfare luck*. Reflection
and discussion can help to identify possible improvements for future similar cases.
In particular, there is benefit in evaluating how well one has achieved behaviour
changes in oneself. There are many things one can test, including one's empathy,
clinical reasoning and communication skills. However, it should be remembered
that communication is *good* or *bad* (only) insofar as it is *effective* (Tate 2003). The
same applies for all veterinary work – the ultimate measure should be whether we
are achieving our welfare goals.

Summary and key recommendations

- We can prevent, cure or palliate feelings and their causes. There is a danger of focusing on
  symptoms without considering the underlying feelings. We can minimise iatrogenic harms
  by refinements such as analgesia, good handling and environmental enrichment and
  avoiding unpleasant interactions.
- We can alter owners' behaviours through legal methods such as refusing to give
  overtreatment or reporting them to authorities, economic methods such as pro bono
  treatment and identifying *win-win* options, and communicative methods using insights from
  human medical communication skills and social marketing to involve and engage the owner
  through *their* decision-making steps using joint decision-making and participatory methods.
  We can guide them through building blocks and small steps, and identify barriers and
  benefits to them. We can use our own authority as *key opinion leaders*, vet–client relations,
  personal appeals and comparison to owners' peers.
- We can also affect colleagues and ourselves through similar methods, by aiming for better
  communication, coordination and collaboration, and identification of barriers and benefits,
  in order to maximise our *welfare efficiency*.

Selected further reading

Communication skills within human medicine by Silverman *et al.* (2005), Myerscough and Ford (1996) and Lloyd and Bor (2004), and within veterinary medicine by Adams and Frankel (2007). Communication with paediatric patients' parents are described by Laing (1996). Ideas to increase compliance are given by Wayner and Heinke (2006). Narrative methods are discussed by Tovey (1998), Hudson Jones (1998), Greenhalgh and Hurwitz (1998) and Charon (2006). Social marketing is reviewed by McKenzie-Mohr and Smith (1999). A good book of participatory tools used in other context is International HIV/AIDS Alliance 2006.

Veterinary economics are discussed by Mosteller (2008) and the welfare implications by Yeates (2012d). Hard selling is discussed by Main (2006), clinical governance by SPVS (2007) and whistle-blowing by Yeates (2012c), while Taylor *et al.* (2007) review the Health Belief Model.

Beyond the Clinic

6

6.1 Beyond Patients

Chapters 1 to 5 have focused on ways to improve our welfare accounts by helping our patients. We can also add value to our veterinary work, and improve our welfare accounts, by looking beyond our patients to *other* animals. As with pathological diseases, veterinary practitioners can spread *welfare contagion*. This can be a bad thing when welfare-unfriendly practices (e.g. anachronistic advice or inappropriate animal handling methods) become endemic in a veterinary clinic, which then becomes a source of infection of newly graduated veterinary professionals and owners. But clinics can also spread good practices, and this is arguably part of their role in society. We can work as a profession to inform and motivate society (Sections 6.4 to 6.9), or go beyond our clients in our local areas (discussed in Sections 6.2 and 6.3). Closer to home, we can spread good practices to our clients while they are in our clinic and help their other animals.

We can advise clients about *future* animals, for example by giving prophylactic advice when clients are considering purchasing another animal or breeding their own animals. We can proactively advise on husbandry, since owners may be likely to purchase equipment before or while they obtain the animal. We can also try to persuade them to obtain multiple gregarious animals before they get just one (and advise about introducing new animals or choosing pre-bonded pairs) or to obtain a single non-gregarious animal before they get several.

Even better, we can give advice on what animal to get, by informing purchasers about what things to think about, what to look for in the animal and what questions

Animal Welfare in Veterinary Practice, First Edition. James Yeates and Sean Wensley.
© 2013 Universities Federation for Animal Welfare. Published 2013 by Blackwell Publishing Ltd.

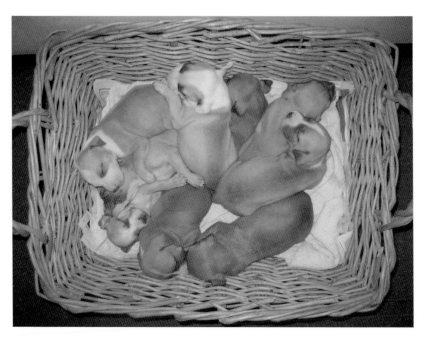

Figure 6.1   Pre-purchase advice may avoid later relinquishment or abandonment. (Courtesy of RSPCA Bristol.)

to ask the seller (e.g. vaccination and health status, health tests and personality). We can advise owners on their choice of species, breed, age and source, and inform them about breed-related conditions and possible medical costs and lifestyle compatibility. We can also help owners to decide whether to get an animal at all, and to check they have everything needed to look after an animal. This advice may be structured around the acronym "PETS" – place, exercise, time and spend (PDSA 2010).

Pre-purchase veterinary advice can help clients to have more realistic expectations and better owner–animal relationships (Kidd *et al.* 1992; Serpell 1996), and evidence (e.g. Patronek *et al.* 1996; New *et al.* 2000; Scarlett *et al.* 2002) also suggests such advice may make it less likely the owner will relinquish the animal into rescue shelters (Figure 6.1). Veterinary professionals may also reduce relinquishment by suggesting people rehome pets rather than buy deliberately bred animals and advising neutering to prevent animals being bred for whom there are not available good homes.

This advice can spread as further contagion. Owners may discuss matters with fellow animal purchasers (e.g. other people looking to buy a puppy or to set up a hobby farm). Purchases may lead to trends where people follow their peers (and buy *status*, fashion or *designer* pets), or copy their parents (and buy the breeds with which they were brought up). Breeders and dealers may respond to consumer demand for animals who are set up for better lives (e.g. by being socialised or already in a bonded pair). Changing owners' decisions can therefore have much wider *ripple effects* on future purchasers.

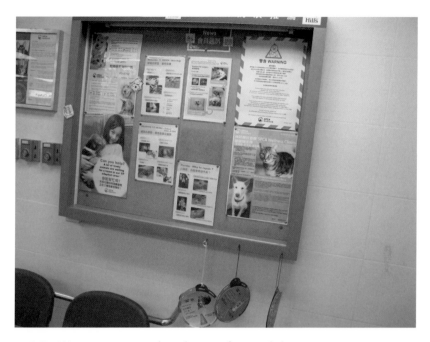

Figure 6.2 Waiting room noticeboards can inform and direct owners to improve animals' welfare. (Courtesy of SPCA Hong Kong.)

Clinics who want to give this advice may need to be proactive about getting owners into the surgery to discuss issues. Most practices can think of effective methods (advertising, special offers, etc.) and the benefits (increased footfall, future bonded clients, etc.), but may also be concerned with the perceived barriers. Practices can minimise potential barriers such as staffing costs, for example by scheduling pre-purchase consults on afternoons when staff are otherwise less busy; charging pre-purchase consultation fees, which are reimbursed if the clients come to you for their first vaccination; or include free pre-purchase advice within an overall (cradle-to-the-grave) health package. Plus, giving such advice can save time overall by preventing the need for later (usually long and uncharged) discussions of behavioural problems.

We can help other animals by being general *animal welfare ambassadors* to our clients. This uses our direct personal contact with many people and our status as key opinion leaders on animal welfare issues. Waiting room noticeboards can advertise only breeders who the practice knows are responsible (e.g. who come to the practice to obtain the appropriate health tests) and trainers the practice knows use appropriate methods (e.g. are registered with a recommended body, avoid aversive training or still propagating dominance-based theories). Noticeboards can also provide targeted welfare advice (Figure 6.2). This leadership can be especially contagious when veterinary professionals advise clients who are also key opinion leaders, such as prominent farmers, breeders, trainers or celebrities.

This advocacy can go beyond the species we treat. Farm animal practitioners can advise farmers about the welfare of other animals (e.g. their sheepdogs). Small animal practitioners can advise pet owners about the welfare of animals that produce their food, and encourage owners to purchase higher welfare farm products. Many clients do not understand farming and distance themselves from thinking about it (Frewer & Salter 2002; McEarchern & Schroeder 2002), so we can help to inform, remind and inspire people about farm animal welfare. Opportunities are surprisingly common. For example, we can mention welfare issues in discussions about bland diets (e.g. chicken) or training (e.g. sausages and other treats). Some practices even put posters or leaflets in the waiting room. Our knowledge of client decision-making, and our experience in delivering complex scientific information to laypeople, can help us to deliver messages appropriately and tailor them to each client. For example, rather than explaining the complexities of Chapters 1, 3 and 4, we can instead advise on *small steps* owners can feasibly implement, such as using only certain shops. Where we feel we lack this knowledge, our professional bodies or trustworthy charities can provide accessible resources we can adapt.

6.2 Beyond Clients

We may also want to act as *animal welfare ambassadors* to non-clients. Veterinary professionals are especially well placed to do this. We are experienced at communicating problems in understandable, non-emotive language. We have credibility and authority as key opinion leaders, so our letters or emails can carry significant weight. We can also often provide practical solutions to make the messages more constructive and effective.

Veterinary practices can forge relationships with other local key opinion formers such as foot-trimmers, nutritionists, artificial insemination technicians, breeders, trainers, riding schools and instructors, racetracks, groomers, boarding kennels and shops. For example, collaborating with pet shops can allow you to educate staff on how to care for stock and advise pet purchasers, perhaps providing jointly branded advice leaflets with your logo and address. We can also write to retailers (e.g. pet shops or grocers), businesses (e.g. zoological gardens), local authorities and politicians about issues of concern.

Some motivated practices also do local charity work, such as free health checks or microchipping (Figure 6.3). These can act as advertising and increase footfall, and can be easy to organise by linking them to national programmes which provide literature, administrative and media support. Other practices put on community events or visit local groups such as schools, children's clubs and learned societies.

Veterinary professionals can highlight welfare messages through the local media (e.g. local newspapers and radio), social media (e.g. blogging or networking sites) or specialist media (e.g. farming or equine magazines). We can report individual cases (e.g.

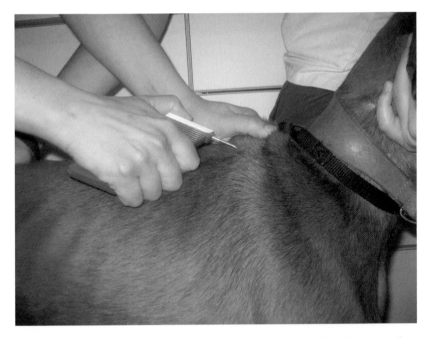

Figure 6.3 Welfare-focused practices can do local charity work such as free microchipping. (Courtesy of SPCA Hong Kong.)

a stick injury), case series (e.g. an increased incidence of digital dermatitis) or general issues (e.g. biosecurity). Good cases may be those that are unusual, topical, human and relevant to the audience – news stories are not always about scandal, celebrity and money – and which come with good pictures and personal quotations. Good cases should also relate to animal welfare issues that readers can do something to prevent (e.g. parvovirus or fishing-line injuries). For example, some cases highlight the harmfulness of common practices such as fireworks and balloon races (Figure 6.4). Media work can provide free marketing, improve the practice's reputation for compassion, be enjoyable, improve morale, reduce future frustrations and provide excellent opportunities for welfare offsetting. The risk of being misquoted or misreported is actually a very low risk because reporters want to maintain good relationships and obtain heart-warming stories. Some practices add value by scheduling perennial stories (e.g. firework fears) and running competitions asking readers to vote for their favourite story.

6.3 Professional Cooperation

Another way to achieve welfare improvements is for local practices to work together. Cooperation can take three forms: coordination, communication and collaboration. Welfare standards can be contagious within the profession as much as they are in the wider society.

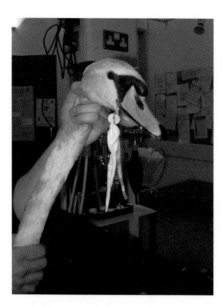

Figure 6.4 Good stories are often topical and have a real welfare message, such as highlighting the dangers of balloon races.(Courtesy of RSPCA Bristol.)

Coordination involves practices cooperating to harmonise their work to best improve animal welfare. For example, if local practices agree not to provide a particular overtreatment (e.g. bulldog caesarians without neutering), owners will not have the option of selecting different practices without travelling long distances – so practices avoid the *race to the bottom* driven by non-cooperative competition.

Even where coordination is not possible due to legal barriers or inter-practice politics, there is still benefit to better inter-practice *communication* about welfare-relevant issues, cases and practice policies. Such communication can mutually educate each practice with fresh and outside ideas and solutions, and knowing what other practices do can help to decide whether tactical overtreatment is appropriate.

Even better is where practices enter into *collaboration* to work together on an issue. Practices might share stock that is rarely used but urgently needed or expensive equipment and facilities. Others may collaborate on specific projects, such as obtaining and storing blood banks or donor registers, organising continuing professional development sessions on animal welfare topics or staging joint community events.

Cooperation can also be beneficial at the level of the whole profession. This cooperation can also involve communication, coordination and collaboration, through both regulatory and membership-based professional bodies.

Communication within the profession can help to discuss ideas and disseminate information. It can help people to identify priorities and share new or good practices. It can also help veterinary professionals to give each other an idea of the prevalent social norms, which they can use as a benchmark in their decision-making.

Coordination within the profession can harmonise and organise practices on a national scale. Many countries have codes of practice or deontologies that describe veterinary professional responsibilities, enforced by regulatory and disciplinary committees that can remove a professional's licence to practise. These may describe general principles or specific duties, such as prohibiting certain interventions or specifying conditions under which interventions may be performed (e.g. that kidney transplants may be performed only by specialist teams). Countries can also set practice standards, enforced through inspection and accreditation, to promote higher standards of care.

Professional regulation can help to address issues that create difficult dilemmas for individual veterinary practitioners. Banning the routine prescription of coccidiostats means the only option is for farmers to improve their husbandry. Banning feline declawing and canine vocal cord resection means owners cannot purchase an animal and then force the veterinary professional to choose between obliging the client or euthanasing the animal. Banning killing animals without a *reasonable reason* could mean owners do not see their animals as disposable. Banning overtreatment means owners cannot go to a less scrupulous practice. These rules would cause welfare problems until owners realise that the easy option is prohibited, but they can have beneficial effects in the long term. Where dilemmas continue, professional regulation can also mandate welfare offsetting in certain situations (such as reporting conformation-altering surgeries).

We are often reluctant for professional bodies to have any power over our clinical decisions. However, in some cases we might welcome professional regulation. Sometimes not having one option can *empower* us not to provide (or offer) welfare-unfriendly options, by providing an argument to clients (that we are not allowed), reducing perceived legal risks (as a legal defence for not doing something) and reducing the pressure to provide a treatment competitors provide (by preventing them from doing so). Even where restrictions of clinical autonomy do restrict the beneficial use of a treatment, this restriction may often be worth the benefit of restricting *misuse*, so restrictions may be beneficial overall even if some cases would benefit from an option being permitted. For example, banning congenital hernia repair without neutering could mean some breeders choose not to get the operation done, but this ban could also help to prevent hereditary problems being passed on. Similarly, banning electronic shock collars (ESCs) may be beneficial even if they are useful in some cases.

Alternatively, professional bodies can provide guidelines that, like *standard operating procedures* (SOPs), can be recommendations which allow practitioners to deviate in exceptional cases (but need to be prepared to defend that deviation). Another solution is to create clinical ethics committees, either nationally or in each university or practice, which could review specific cases similar to equivalent systems that are increasingly common in human hospitals and animal research institutions. A more general approach is for codes to mandate very general duties that can be interpreted by disciplinary committees. This would allow regulatory bodies to make general rules such as prohibiting overtreatment or requiring that practitioners provide *reasonable* emergency treatment.

Many countries also have veterinary oaths that graduates swear on entering the profession. Professional codes and oaths often focus on duties to colleagues and clients, based on the old rationales for the veterinary profession described in Section 1.2, but it is important that they are increasingly based on what is best for animal welfare. For example, the American Veterinary Medical Association has recently updated its oath to include a stronger animal welfare commitment. These promises are usually taken to prescribe how veterinary professionals behave in their work, but oaths should not only apply from 8 am to 7 pm – a promise to make animal welfare one's main consideration should apply to one's whole life.

6.4 Professional Collaboration

We can also collaborate as a profession. As a profession, we have a greater capacity to work on the bigger picture than we do individually or locally. Professional bodies may have greater power to lobby governments, to engage industries, to fund or coordinate research to contribute to the media. They also can draw on the authority and trust individual members of society have for individual members of the profession, so that the professional bodies are a credible community leader on a national or international level. Professional bodies (and their officers) have their own animal welfare accounts. Professional collaboration also helps its members by helping us fulfil our claims that we are *welfare experts* and *animal advocates*, and ensuring that we remain centrally involved in animal welfare issues.

Professional bodies need to make decisions, and this can draw on the same principles as our clinical decision-making. In both cases, we need to be welfare-focused, we need to be reflective and effective, we need to realistically consider the constraints and barriers, we need to engage the relevant people and we need to use knowledge, empathy and reasoning. The processes are also similar. Professional bodies need to make assessments and decisions, and these involve a similar five steps (Figure 6.5).

Steps 1 to 3 lead to an assessment of welfare issues. This can be a position statement that informs or advises members or other people. These positions can assess situations and highlight the importance of welfare problems, or they can evaluate the options that are available. They are equivalent to evaluations in clinical decision-making and involve similar steps.

Step 1 involves identifying issues. Sometimes this is done by our members, and we can feed into our professional bodies' decision-making processes. In other cases, issues are highlighted by public concern, such as when a law is being discussed or an issue hits the media. Steps 2 and 3 involve interpretation and evaluation. As for clinical assessments, these need to utilise both science and our experiences. We need to utilise science in our decisions wherever possible, because of its importance in resolving reaching objective assessments.

The veterinary profession is also well placed to make decisions where scientific *proof* is lacking. Other bodies have a difficult choice about what to do when science

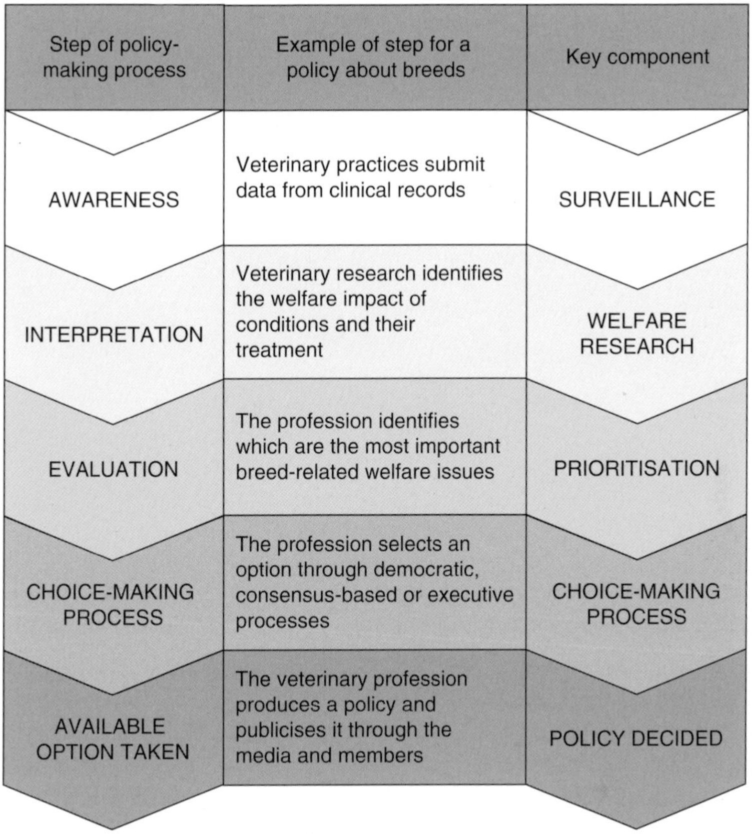

Step of policy-making process	Example of step for a policy about breeds	Key component
AWARENESS	Veterinary practices submit data from clinical records	SURVEILLANCE
INTERPRETATION	Veterinary research identifies the welfare impact of conditions and their treatment	WELFARE RESEARCH
EVALUATION	The profession identifies which are the most important breed-related welfare issues	PRIORITISATION
CHOICE-MAKING PROCESS	The profession selects an option through democratic, consensus-based or executive processes	CHOICE-MAKING PROCESS
AVAILABLE OPTION TAKEN	The veterinary profession produces a policy and publicises it through the media and members	POLICY DECIDED

Figure 6.5 Model of policy-making process for professional bodies.

is lacking. They can remain silent unless there is *sufficient* evidence, but risk seeming weak, indecisive, dishonest or disingenuous (e.g. using the lack of science to delay decisions or maintain the status quo). Alternatively, they can make bold statements without evidence, but risk being criticised for being unreliable and unobjective. We can avoid both risks because our clinical training hones our skills at making assessments even without directly applicable science. Our professional bodies can draw on members' practical experience and general understanding of biology (Figure 6.6), and thus avoid inactivity when there is a lack of data. For example, many practitioners are *situated* in the context of the issue, who thereby see welfare problems and interventions first-hand.

As well as situated practitioners' views, our professional bodies' position-making should draw on the expert knowledge of the specialists within our profession. While veterinary professionals can be considered animal welfare experts relative to the public, there are animal welfare specialists within the profession with an even greater degree of specific knowledge and experience. Veterinary animal welfare

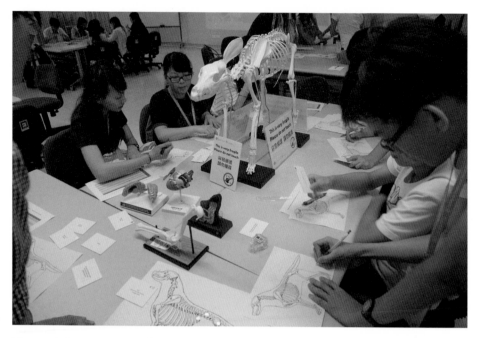

Figure 6.6 Veterinary professionals can draw on their wide general knowledge of animals' biology. (Courtesy of Royal Veterinary College, Hong Kong Ltd.)

experts can be more easily identified since the recent establishment of a European College of Animal Welfare and Behavioural Medicine. There are also animal welfare experts outside the profession. The opinions of these experts can – and often should – carry greater weight than those of non-specialists. Just as we respect the opinions of specialists in medicine and immunology when making policies about vaccination, so can more respect be afforded to the views of those with a proven animal welfare specialisation, who devote considerable time, effort and learning to the subject of animal welfare. Nevertheless, welfare experts' opinions should be based on *building blocks* of information provided by situated practitioners, even if the welfare experts make the overall assessment.

Steps 4 and 5 lead to a recommendation for action on the part of the professional body itself. This can be a policy, which is something the professional body intends to do. Some policies may be internally focused, such as where to buy food for catering or how to regulate members. Others may be externally focused, such as how to drive legislative or societal change. These policies then need to be converted into actions, in order to achieve animal welfare improvements. Step 5 involves actually fulfilling those intentions. Our policies need to be effective. Sometimes, this means we need to balance idealism and realism. We may need to suggest *small steps* that help take society on a journey.

6.5 Professional Barriers and Biases

As for clinical decision-making, we need to minimise and avoid potential problems in each step of professional bodies' policy-making. In Step 1, we may identify issues inappropriately. We may focus on issues only reactively when they are topical in the news or subject to government consultations. Reactive work helps us maintain our reputation as a source of opinion on welfare issues. Similarly, issues raised by our members can be unavoidably skewed; for example, situated practitioners may see some issues more commonly (e.g. those that require veterinary interventions) but not others (e.g. mutilations we authorise but do not perform). Ideally, issues for consideration should be raised by more objective methods, based on welfare surveillance, as discussed in Section 6.6.

During Step 2, we may misinterpret issues for several reasons. Decisions may be made by a minority of us who happen to sit on relevant councils or committees, who may be non-practising (and therefore less exposed) or less recently graduated (and perhaps therefore less up to date). Decisions made by situated practitioners can also be biased due to our habituation or hardening to things we see or perform regularly (e.g. to breed-related conditions, systemic on-farm problems or post-operative pain). For some subjects, most veterinary professionals have not had the opportunity (or time) to consider in depth. For example, the average veterinary professional may have limited knowledge about cephalopods' neural system, cognitive capabilities or capacity to feel pain. More objective interpretations can be based on scientific information, although an overreliance on science may make us overly conservative. One solution is to obtain evidence through veterinary animal welfare research, as discussed in Section 6.7. Another solution is to use our expert opinion within the profession, for example in an expert animal welfare committee.

In Step 3, our professional bodies may risk inaccurate evaluations. Importantly, we may inappropriately transfer our clinical assessments concerning individual cases to our wider assessments concerning the big-picture. As practitioners, we must consider the wider economic and legal situations as unchangeable constraints. As professional bodies, we must also consider whether these constraints can be changed by wider action. For example, practitioners may assess ESCs as being beneficial for some pets, but this does not entail that allowing ESCs is beneficial on a national level if banning ESCs would help more animals than it would harm (e.g. if ESCs are frequently used on many animals inappropriately) or if a ban would lead to other progressive changes (e.g. better fencing or use of more positive training methods). Professional bodies can avoid these dangers by giving more sophisticated and conditional answers. For example, we can conclude that a mutilation should be allowed if current intensive farming methods are allowed to continue, but that it would be better if sufficient support were given to improving general husbandry standards.

Table 6.1 Key principles for veterinary policy-making and their effect on proactivity.

Principles that may promote inactivity	Principles that may promote proactivity
Consistency	Idealism
Focus	Integrity
Neutrality	Forthrightness
Practicality	Meaningfulness
Reliability	Progressive

When choosing what they are going to do in Step 4, professional bodies' policy-making has to balance a number of different values and we may excessively focus on some more than others. For example, some values can drive us towards proactivity, others towards inactivity or reactivity (Table 6.1). For example, a desire to maintain our reliability makes us wary of saying anything that might be challenged as incorrect or biased, which may bias us towards providing only conservative statements (or none at all). At the same time, such reticence can open professional bodies (and especially their officers) to criticism. For example, inactivity can make us seem complicit in the status quo (Waldau 2011), especially if we remain silent while claiming to be advocates. We need to combine practice advocacy with a solid basis – but it is a challenge to judge how proactive and how solid.

Finally, in Step 5, another potential barrier for professional bodies – as for practitioners – is its limited resources. Researching, debating and achieving welfare improvements take time and effort, and trying to do too much can risk the profession spreading its resources too thinly or weakening the impact of key messages. There are three main solutions to this.

The first is to use the members. In many professional bodies, only a relatively small percentage of members are actively involved, and most have a limited number of staff. But they have larger numbers of members who, if they are provided with information and engaged, can act as *vectors* and pass on contagious messages using the personal relationships they have with their clients. This makes veterinary welfare education especially important, as discussed in Section 6.8. As individual members, we can also help our professional body to develop and propagate animal welfare positions and policies. Where members are needed to fulfil policies, it is important for us to aim for a professional consensus. Like achieving concordance, this requires engaging members, good communication and open discussions. Consensus can also be built up from agreed building blocks, for example agreeing to focus on animals' feelings, and on what policy-making processes to use, such as specific assessment methods, Delphi processes, elected officers or appointed expert committees.

The second is for us to collaborate with other welfare-focused bodies, such as industry partners, charities, government and non-governmental organisations. In some cases, these other bodies may have the resources but not the authority, so collaboration can be a valuable partnership. One recent success story is the banning of wild bird importation into the European Union, which involved a collaboration between the Royal Society for the Protection of Birds, the RSPCA, the World Parrot Trust, the British Veterinary Association, the Federation of Veterinarians in Europe, alongside other charities and medical experts.

The third is to prioritise our resources. Table 6.2 gives some factors by which bodies should prioritise (which could be evaluated qualitatively or quantitatively). We can focus on the most important animal welfare issues and those we can do most about. We can also focus on specifically *veterinary* responsibilities and accountabilities, or those where improvements can avoid members' welfare dilemmas or offset members' welfare harms. For example, veterinary professional bodies may focus on the avoidance of breed-related conditions that are propagated by veterinary practice, or on the employment of the 3Rs (replacement, refinement and reduction) in the use of animals for toxicology testing of veterinary medicines.

All of these steps need to be combined into one process. An example is given for tackling broiler breeder issues in Table 6.3.

6.6 Veterinary Welfare Surveillance

As for clinical decision-making, policy-making requires an assessment of the welfare issues. Firstly, the profession needs to identify issues through welfare surveillance, such as epidemiological research or widespread audit of welfare issues. Welfare surveillance is equivalent to screening for individual cases, insofar as it demonstrates the extent of welfare issues without interpreting what they mean for the animals. As for individual cases, surveillance can also screen for side effects when policies are implemented. In addition, data can highlight a problem through the media and to politicians.

Welfare surveillance can survey the prevalence of causes and symptoms of welfare problems. These need not only focus on infectious pathological causes, but could also focus on behavioural issues (e.g. Bradshaw *et al.* 2002; Blackwell *et al.* 2005) or anthropogenic causes such as fishing-line injuries (Figure 6.7). Welfare surveillance can also look for population-level indicators, such as the extent of owners' knowledge about how to care for their animal (e.g. PDSA 2011) or the number and nature of state veterinary inspections (e.g. RSPCA 2008). Further research can investigate the causes of those causes, such as epidemiological analysis to determine disease risk factors or sociological research to examine human behaviours, for example looking at the best ways to communicate information about welfare issues (e.g. Yeates *et al.* 2011). Surveys can examine how severe welfare issues are perceived to be by veterinary professionals (e.g. Yeates and Main 2011a).

Table 6.2 Factors for professional bodies to consider when prioritising issues/actions.

Factor	Examples
Animal welfare importance	Intensity for animals affected (average and range)
	Duration and frequency for animals affected (average and range)
	Numbers of animals affected
	Confidence in knowledge about the issue
External effects	Effects on other animals
	Effects on humans
	Effects on the environment
Responsibility	The extent to which the welfare issue was caused by humans
	The extent to which the welfare issue was caused by veterinary professionals (offsetting)
	The extent to which the veterinary profession has a moral responsibility for those animals
	The extent to which the veterinary profession has a legal responsibility for those animals
Exigency	Relative urgency of the issue (i.e. does something need doing now or can it wait)
Benefits to the profession	Direct benefits to the profession (e.g. financial)
	Indirect benefits to the profession (e.g. political, image)
	Likelihood action will facilitate further action in the future
Importance for professional body's members	Importance to members (demonstrated by input into professional policy-making)
	Direct benefits to the profession in achieving members' welfare goals
	Direct benefits to the profession in avoiding dilemmas
	Indirect benefits to the profession (e.g. financial benefits or increased respect)
	Indirect costs to members (e.g. loss of revenue)
Barriers for the profession	Direct costs to the profession (e.g. time, resources)
	Indirect costs to the profession (e.g. reputation)
	Opportunity costs of doing something about it (in terms of weakening ability to do something about other issues)
Actions and responsibilities of other parties	Likelihood other people will achieve the changes instead and/or better unassisted
	Long-term benefits in cooperation (e.g. political)
Feasibility of tackling the problem	Ability of the profession to perform desired action
	Probability of action having an effect
	Extent of effect in reducing severity, duration, frequency and numbers
Procedural elements	Representation of members' inputs through the body's decision-making processes

Table 6.3 How the veterinary profession might help tackle broiler breeder welfare.

Step, activity and outcome	Examples
Step 1	**Identify welfare issues – surveillance**
Utilise existing research to identify issues	Growth rate has increased significantly through breeding (Havenstein *et al.* 2003)
	Effect of selection for fast growth on anatomy and physiology of broilers (Bessei 2006)
	Feed restriction of breeders, e.g. from 14 weeks (Hocking *et al.* 1989)
	Quantitative restriction, e.g. 20–25% of ad lib intake (Mench 2002), increasing towards peak lay (Hocking 1996)
	Some breeders fed every other day (Mench 1988)
	Other breeds may require less or no feed restriction (Whitehead *et al.* 1987)
Carry out surveillance through veterinary practitioners	Qualitative survey to ask broiler-industry-situated practitioners qualitative perceptions
	Quantitative retrospective study using broiler-industry-situated practitioners' clinical notes
	Quantitative prospective study with broiler-industry-situated practitioners' recording findings
Outcome: List of issues	**Broiler breeder starvation, de-beaking, dubbing, lameness, etc.**
Step 2	**Interpret welfare issues**
Collect available scientific research that may help assess the issues identified	Relate dietary restriction to quality, quantity and behavioural needs (Kasanen *et al.* 2010)
	Identify link of starvation to *frustration-behaviours*, e.g. spot-pecking stereotypies, polydipsia and voracious feeding (Koštál *et al.* 1992; Savory *et al.* 1992, 1993a,b, Hocking 1993, 1996, Savory and Maros 1993, Hocking, *et al.* 2001)
	Feed restriction associated with elevated cortisol (Maxwell *et al.* 1990, 1992; Hocking *et al.* 1993, 1996, 2001; Savory and Maros 1993, Savory *et al.* 1993a,b)
	Ad lib feeding can lead to vaginal prolapse, heart failure and lameness (Savory *et al.* 1993b), increased aggression (Millman & Duncan 2000), and decreased immune function (O'sullivan *et al.* 1991; Hocking *et al.* 1996)
	Feed restriction associated with higher mortality (Hocking *et al.* 2002)
	Motivation to feed may vary between individuals (Savory *et al.* 1993a, Savory & Mann 1999; Savory & Lariviere 2000)
	Lame broiler chickens self-select analgesic (Danbury *et al.* 2000)

(Continued)

Table 6.3 *(Cont'd)*

Step, activity and outcome	Examples
Collect scientists' interpretations	Overall assessments of welfare issue (Julian 2005; Renema *et al.* 2007; SCAHAW 2000)
	Stereotypies may represent coping methods (Koštál *et al.* 1992; Savory *et al.* 1992, 1993b)
	Ad lib feeding leads to worse biological function (Hocking *et al.* 1993, 1996, 2001)
Commission or conduct research	Preference studies about how broiler breeders choose between hunger and pain
Use expert opinion	Broiler-industry-situated and poultry specialists consider higher egg-production better welfare
	Animal welfare specialists conclude:
	• Elevated cortisol and decreased immune function to signify stress due to hunger and frustration
	• Lameness to signify pain
	• Vaginal prolapsed and heart failure to cause malaise and pain
Outcome: Interpretation of issues	**Conclude that broiler breeders suffer hunger or pain**
Step 3	**Evaluation**
Use scientific data	Allowing animals to forage may reduce the negative hunger experiences (Robert *et al.* 1997; De Leeuw & Ekkel 2004)
	Signs of frustration occur on all feeding methods (Savory *et al.* 1996; Savory & Lariviere 2000; de Jong *et al.* 2005; Hocking 2006)
	Announcing food, to allow anticipation, may improve animal welfare (de Jonge *et al.* 2008)
Use scientists' evaluations	Where welfare is maximised at around 60% of ad lib intake (Hocking 2004)
Use other bodies' evaluations	EFSA reports (Decuypere *et al.* 2006)
Outcome: Produce position statement	**Produce position statement**
Step 4	**Choice-making**
Utilise others' suggestions	Apply/adapt published opinions (eg Brillard 2001)
Determine foundational building blocks	Concern for broiler breeders' feelings
Determine policymaking process	Using expert committee
Outcome: Produce policy	**Produce policy**
Step 5	**Achieve policy**
Prioritise issues	e.g. to focus on broiler breeders instead of fish, parasites, etc.
Collaboration	Consider working with other bodies
Use members	Consider empowering members with advice to write to local retailers, press and politicians
Prioritise methods	Decide most effective method to effect change
Outcome: Activity	**Implement priority actions**

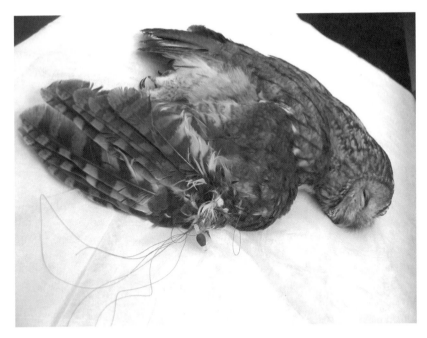

Figure 6.7 Veterinary welfare surveillance can survey issues caused by human practices such as fishing-line injuries to non-target species. (Courtesy of RSPCA Bristol.)

Veterinary professionals at the front line are valuable sources of information for welfare surveillance, through our direct, personal, frequent and meaningful contact with many animals and their owners, with frequent discussions about welfare issues (Shaw *et al.* 2004). Surveys and data-mining from clinical notes can usefully estimate the prevalence of problems (e.g. the prevalence of breed-related conditions or some mutilations), and veterinary practitioners can provide assessments of the severity of the issues they see.

There are difficulties within welfare surveillance, similar to those within welfare assessment. When reporting, we may inaccurately assess welfare problems (as for individual patients), and those in unblinded studies may even give biased responses (e.g. to reflect themselves positively or to drive policy). The patients presented to veterinary practices may not be representative of the animal population as a whole, insofar as patients may receive above average care from their owners, because more caring owners will seek more veterinary advice (Slater *et al.* 2008) or because veterinary advice can improve subsequent care (Patronek *et al.* 1996; c.f. Salman *et al.* 1998). These problems create a temptation to obtain information that is easily measured, rather than what is most useful. Unfortunately, inaccurate information can be misleading, as well as diverting resources from better surveillances. Some badly done surveys are little more than publicity stunts. Good welfare surveillance should use the same criteria described in Box 5.5.

Interpreting and evaluating welfare surveillance data is even more complicated than assessing an individual patient's welfare. It can require comparisons across different types of welfare issues, across causes of welfare issues and across individuals and species. Different species respond to circumstances in different ways and may not experience the same feelings in comparable contexts. For example, different species may vary in their sensitivities to pain, behavioural signs, anatomies, psychological needs and experience of time. Nevertheless, where such comparisons need to be made, these controversies need solving.

There are many areas where we can benefit from more research. As examples, more welfare surveillance is needed to identify the incidence of breed-related conditions (and recent years have seen this point made about pedigree dogs in particular); the husbandry methods of companion animals, horses and hobby farm animals; owners' understanding of welfare issues; how much information veterinary professionals provide about welfare issues and how many animals are euthanased for avoidable problems. For all such issues, surveillance needs to continue, in order to monitor the effects of interventions (e.g. whether changes in dog breeding have any negative effects) and comparative studies can identify which policies or activities actually lead to the most welfare improvements.

Although more research is often valuable, this does not always mean that nothing can be done until the research is done. There is a temptation for policy-makers and industries to maintain the status quo, or to permit a potentially harmful practice, until there is *sufficient* research to evidence its harmfulness. This may be especially likely when people have vested interests in continuing the practice. The veterinary profession can provide authoritative advice in the absence of scientific information.

6.7 Veterinary Welfare Research

Veterinary research helps us to interpret identified welfare issues, both for clinical decision-making and for professional policy-making. Veterinary research has always been an important role of the veterinary profession, and most veterinary students are exposed to veterinary scientists and scientific methods. Research findings provide an evidence-base for interpretation and choice-making, challenge or support established methods and validate or refute new hypotheses. Engaging in research can afford practitioners a good means of welfare offsetting, and may even improve the level of care, based on the *Hawthorne effect* in which research subjects improve their work when they are in an experiment (Ducrot *et al.* 1998; Mangione-Smith *et al.* 1999).

Veterinary research has historically investigated health-related issues – the same issues on which veterinary practice has focused. We have usually investigated pathological conditions, using pathophysiological measures such as routine biochemistry, anatomical measurements, functional assessments (e.g. gait), some

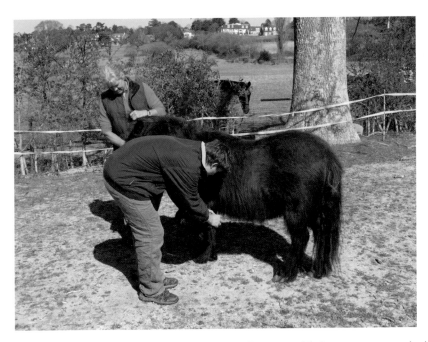

Figure 6.8 Clinical parameters should be gathered as part of holistic assessments, both in practice and in research. (Courtesy of James Yeates.)

behavioural symptoms (e.g. lameness) and longevity. These are useful measures of important causes and symptoms of animal welfare, but can mislead decision-making if they are not applied as part of a holistic assessment (Figure 6.8). For example, a scientific report could promote overtreatment by measuring median survival time and not assessing quality-of-life. As veterinary practice becomes more aware of non-health aspects of animal welfare, this is being paralleled by veterinary research becoming increasingly welfare-focused. This increasingly allows practitioners to make evidence-based decisions about other welfare issues.

One way in which our veterinary research can become more welfare-focused is if we study health issues using non-health welfare assessment parameters. In some cases, these measures can be more directly related to animals' feelings (e.g. "return to pain-free function"). Studies can also provide us with more holistic assessments of the animal's welfare by combining multiple parameters into an overall assessment, or by using overall assessments such as owner-rated quality-of-life. Some of these are quite complicated and subjective measures, but sometimes the more complicated and subjective parameters are more directly important from a welfare perspective. Subjective assessments may be especially justified in case reports that describe how individual animals experienced the condition, since non-representativeness is in the nature of case reports.

Many veterinary studies combine traditional pathophysiological measures with other welfare parameters. This combination provides a wider insight into welfare problems and improvements. It also helps to elucidate the relationships between pathophysiological and other welfare parameters. For example, a study that looked at the effect of a drug on plasma urea and creatinine *and* overall welfare would give information about (a) the drug's effect on azotaemia, (b) the drug's effect on welfare and also (c) the relationship between azotaemia and overall welfare. Understanding this relationship helps practitioners to translate earlier studies that use only traditional parameters into what they mean for a patient's quality-of-life.

Another way in which veterinary research can become more welfare-focused is in producing findings that can be more easily adapted to individual cases. We tend to minimise the effects of inter-individual variations in our studies, but these inter-individual variations are very important when applying scientific evidence to our cases. Studies can help practitioners more by highlighting important inter-individual variations (and attempting to explain those variations). Veterinary research might also be more welfare-focused in helping practitioners to make decisions and achieve animal welfare goals in situations where there are specific constraints or barriers, for example what treatment is best given for different risks of non-compliance. Again, practitioners might find studies more useful if they help us to decide what to do about different clients, or types of clients.

One more way in which our veterinary research can become more welfare-focused is in investigating non-health welfare issues. Clinical trials can evaluate animal welfare assessment and communication methods. Other studies can look at issues of housing, nutrition, company and feelings in conditions not related to pathological problems. These have tended to be part of animal welfare science and not veterinary science, but the former could be considered part of the latter if veterinary science adequately increased its remit. In particular, veterinary science could give greater weight to animal welfare issues within veterinary contexts, such as during hospitalisation (Yeates 2012a).

For some studies, barriers to in-practice research might need to be addressed. Funding limitations can be minimised by using inexpensive behavioural parameters. Legal barriers might be addressed by focusing on retrospective case reports or non-harmful clinical trials if these are allowed without a licence. Practitioners may also be worried about the technical skills required to plan successful studies and write publishable papers. Devising a well-designed experiment to test a hypothesis and analysing the data require aptitude and training. This training may be able to develop the aptitudes created in practice. Designing research questions and methodologies involve developing the abilities to apply hypothetico-deductive and inductive methods that practitioners use in assessing patients' welfare (Fillippich 2000). Publishing involves communication abilities that practitioners use in relating findings to colleagues and clients. Nevertheless, scientific research requires a high level of skill and knowledge, so practitioners may benefit from undertaking specific training, collaborating with experienced researchers (so long as they will commit the necessary time and effort), and from the "Selected further reading" listed later in the text.

6.8 Veterinary Welfare Education

Veterinary education is one way to achieve widespread welfare improvements. It occurs through many agencies, including universities, textbooks, clinical clubs, practice meetings, tea-breaks and social settings. It can be taught by lecturers, university clinicians, residents, supervisors, examiners and all practitioners where they have the ability to inform or influence others. It reaches specialists, non-specialist veterinary professionals, undergraduates, paraprofessionals and members of the public. Many veterinary schools provide dedicated welfare courses as a core part of their undergraduate programmes, usually included within pre-clinical studies. Several countries allow veterinary professionals to specialise in animal welfare, for example through the College of Animal Welfare and Behavioural Medicine Diplomas or UK Royal College of Veterinary Surgeons (RCVS) Certificates in Animal Welfare Science, Ethics and Law.

Education can transfer new and more accurate knowledge, as well as redress erroneous beliefs. Education can increase competences, including technical skills, decision-making skills, communication skills and the skills of applying science to individual cases. These can be combined when veterinary education encourages students to question and reflect upon sources of information, rather than teaching knowledge as unquestionable *scientific facts* to be learnt by rote.

Education can also pass on contagious habits, values and attitudes. This contagion probably occurs whether we intend it or not because lecturers cannot avoid inadvertently influencing students in the same way that practitioners influence their clients. This influence may be especially likely on clinical rotations with impressionable younger students, interns and residents. Good teachers can embrace this influence, and actively and openly discuss their welfare concerns, assessments and treatment choices. This gives students opportunities to learn about how their teachers make decisions, and provides them with welfare-focused role models. Animal welfare teaching may also engender a welfare-focused culture amongst both staff and students.

Since influencing students may be unavoidable, teachers must also avoid bad welfare contagion. Teachers should avoid desensitising students or providing negative role models. A diminishing number of lecturers are dismissive of animal welfare. But many teachers find it hard to discuss welfare issues, and thereby effectively provide a role model for ignoring welfare issues. Other teachers appear to represent welfare as a relatively unimportant *add-on* (e.g. listing a disease's welfare implications after its production, management, financial and even aesthetic effects) or describe welfare issues primarily as production management problems for humans (e.g. hens' broodiness, ewes' mis-mothering, pigs' rooting; *vices*). Others

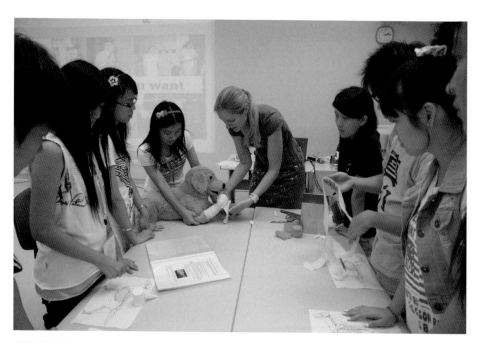

Figure 6.9 Veterinary medical education can use alternatives, such as this model dog. (Courtesy of Royal Veterinary College, Hong Kong Ltd.)

may stress certain elements above others, for example discussing pain more than boredom or frustration.

Education can cause iatrogenic harms to animals within the course, for example in surgery training using live patients under non-terminal anaesthesia, and such harms are now controlled in many countries and there are increasing numbers of good alternatives to animal use (Figure 6.9). More subtly, postgraduate coursework requirements can promote overtreatment by not accepting case reports unless a diagnosis is obtained and a certain type of treatment is given, thereby discouraging clinicians from providing bespoke treatment or euthanasia. Such iatrogenic harms also lead to undesirable welfare contagion, by desensitising students or encouraging overtreatment. Education can also cause wider iatrogenic welfare harms through their recommendations, for example where lectures or textbooks promote overtreatment or suggest overly inflexible protocols that do not allow practitioners to adequately consider each individual patient's welfare. The danger of causing iatrogenic harms may be especially likely in some areas of practice, such as surgery, clinical behavioural therapy, oncology and palliative care, and in pioneering lectures and textbooks in a field that sets precedents for later work.

As well as informing students about animal welfare, education can also encourage engagement and ownership of animal welfare aspects (although there is limited published evidence to support this). Such engagement may be helped by using participatory methods such as case discussions and role playing, which can also develop the teacher's understanding since students, like laypeople, can have valuable insights and complementary understanding of welfare issues. Engagement may also be increased by making the teaching more relevant. Animal welfare lecturers can provide examples of clinical cases to elucidate the implications of welfare concepts.

Clinical teachers can explicitly highlight and discuss animal welfare concepts in their clinical case discussions, especially during in-practice teaching. Some clinicians are nervous about discussing welfare issues. One solution is an anonymous *counselling* service where students can discuss cases with a designated member of staff. However, this solution means students effectively discuss cases behind the clinician's back and without the clinician's input. Contemporaneous discussions involving the clinicians are preferable, but this requires a culture in which students are happy asking questions about patients' welfare and clinicians are comfortable discussing cases. Achieving this requires teaching clinicians about animal welfare, and teaching students communication skills to ask questions tactfully.

6.9 Next Steps

With all this in mind, what can each of us do? Most importantly, all of us can try to always engage in welfare-focused practice. In each case, we should try to make our welfare assessment more accurate and our decision-making more reasoned. We can try to choose the option that is most likely to improve our patients' welfare, not the one that makes us the most money or that makes us feel best (even if owners then do not comply).

We can also try to set aside time to engage in reflective practice. We can reflect on our strengths and weaknesses. We can maintain and extend our knowledge in animal welfare, communication skills and decision-making (even when surgico-medical topics seem more exciting). We can identify and address our barriers and biases and maintain our motivation by keeping the benefits in mind. On busy weeks, this is impossible, but we can use quieter times to step back and reflect.

We can also try to have an effect beyond our everyday practice, especially on issues that we feel frustrated about or which cause us regular dilemmas. We can think of imaginative ways of welfare offsetting and proactively take action to remedy the causes of wider problems that compensate (or overcompensate) for our part in their cause. We can engage with our professional body and animal welfare societies. We can give pro bono time, money or fund-raising efforts to animal welfare charities. We can personally make good consumer choices when we go shopping or to restaurants, so that we embody the welfare standards we want others to emulate.

Hopefully this book has provided some inspiration, encouragement and empowerment to achieve animal welfare improvements in everyday practice and to make a difference in wider welfare issues. The veterinary profession has enormous potential to drive forward change, and effort from individual veterinary professionals has the potential to make a big difference. Changes will not be easy, fast or pleasant. But if veterinary professionals do not drive forward this change, then who will? This is an exciting and pioneering time for us within the animal welfare debate, and ensuring we have a place needs effort from individuals.

This final call to arms leaves the next step for you to decide. Consider what you would like to achieve in the short and long terms, including the possible benefits and barriers, and then plan your own next step. The next step may be a small step such as organising a practice discussion, reading another book on animal welfare, writing a letter to a local paper or summarising your thoughts after this book. It might be more ambitious, such as applying for a course on animal welfare or planning an in-practice research project. What is important is to engage with animal welfare *and* veterinary practice, to make your contribution to the solution and to maximise your animal welfare account.

Summary and key recommendations

- We can take steps beyond our patients and clients to avoid welfare dilemmas and offset the iatrogenic harms we cause. We can be *animal welfare ambassadors* to our clients, so they make better purchasing decisions, and to non-clients through charity work, writing to businesses and politicians, and in the media. We can engage in veterinary welfare surveillance and research, which should combine both pathological and non-pathological welfare parameters. We should provide welfare-focused role models to students and colleagues.
- We can coordinate, communicate and collaborate with other local practices, and as a profession. The profession can also be more proactive, to help members, society and animals. Being overly moderate, over-reliant on science or overly close to the industry can make the profession seem weak or dishonest. We need to maintain our reliability, consistency, neutrality and integrity. We must be realistic and pragmatic, while also being progressive, forthright and idealistic. Policy-making should focus on priorities and should aim for consensus by agreeing transparent building blocks, using situated practitioners, unsituated professionals and animal welfare experts.
- Each of us should choose feasible next steps to improve our welfare accounts by achieving our animal welfare goals.

Selected further reading

The PDSA provides an award-winning website resource to help people choose which species of pet to get, available at www.your-right-pet.org.uk. UFAW is creating a website for genetic diseases of dogs, cats and rabbits to help professionals and owners to make decisions about which breed to get (or not to get) and what advice to give, available at www.ufaw.org.uk/geneticwelfareproblems.php.

Veterinary oaths are discussed by Hewson (2006) and Bones and Yeates (2012), and medics' Hippocratic Oath by Miles (2004). Specialist veterinary animal welfare societies include the UK's Animal Welfare Science, Ethics and Law Veterinary Association (website), the USA's Society for Veterinary Medical Ethics (http://www.svme.org), the American Association of Human-Animal Bond Veterinary professionals (http://aahabv.org) and the Humane Society Veterinary Medical Association (http://www.hsvma.org/). Specialist non-veterinary animal welfare societies include the Universities Federation for Animal Welfare, you country's Society for the Prevention of Cruelty to Animals or international charities such as WSPA (World Society for the Protection of Animals) or CIWF (Compassion in World Farming).

CAWC (2008) discusses animal welfare surveillance. Examples of respondents giving biased ratings to reflect themselves positively are given by Tourangeau and Yan (2007). The *Hawthorne effect* was classically described by Mayo (1933). Mullan *et al.* (2011) provide a good example of improving animal welfare by working with a farming industry. Guidance on research in practice is given by Forbes (2001, 2002) and Holmes and Cockroft (2008), epidemiological research by Thrusfield (1995), statistical advice by Petrie and Watson (1999) and publishing advice by Mason (1995). As specific ideas, qualitative welfare measures are discussed by Verbeke and Viaene (2000) and Velde *et al.* (2002); on combining qualitative and quantitative measures to provide richer explanations by Amaratunga *et al.* (2002) and Johnson and Onwuegbuzie (2004); on Dephi methodologies by Whay *et al.* (2003), Bennett *et al.* (2004) and Collins *et al.* (2009); and on other subjective assessment methods by Meagher (2009). The Hawthorne effect has been demonstrated for human doctors (who prescribe fewer antibiotics for viral infections; Mangione-Smith *et al.* 1999) and farmers (Ducrot *et al.* 1998).

Medical education on communication skills, shared decision-making models and empathy are discussed by Lloyd and King (2004), Latham and Morris (2007), Radford et al. (2003) and Penticuf and Arheart (2005). Veterinary medical education is discussed by Willis *et al.* (2007), Wensley (2008) and other papers in the *Journal of Veterinary Medical Education*. Participatory education is famously proposed and celebrated by Freire (1996). The European College of Animal Welfare and Behavioural Medicine can be investigated at http://www.ebvs.org/component/content/15?task=view&College=ECAWBM, and the RCVS Certificates in Animal Welfare Science, Ethics and Law at http://www.rcvs.org.uk/education/postgraduate-education-for-veterinary-surgeons/certificates/. The WSPA has produced presentations and worksheets for international animal welfare education (2005).

The idea of the veterinary professional within a global profession is discussed by Brown *et al.* (2006).

References

Adams, C.L. & Frankel, R.M. (2007) It may be a dog's life but the relationship with her owners is also key to her health and well being: Communication in veterinary medicine. *Veterinary Clinics of North America: Small Animal Practice*, 37, 1–17.

Ahlstrom, L.A., Mills, P.C. & Mason, K. (2009) Barazone decreases skin lesions and pruritis and increases quality of life in dogs with atopic dermatitis: A blinded, randomised, placebo-controlled trial. *Journal of Veterinary Pharmacology and Therapeutics*, 32, 87–96.

Ainslie, G. (2001) *Breakdown of Will*. Cambridge University Press, Cambridge, UK.

Ajzen, I. (2005) *Attitudes, Personality and Behavior*, 2nd edn. Open University Press, Maidenhead, UK.

Ajzen, I. & Fishbein, M. (1980) *Understanding Attitudes and Predicting Social Behavior*. Prentice-Hall, Englewood Cliffs, NJ.

Albert, A. & Bulcroft, K. (1987) Pets and urban life. *Anthrozoos*, 1, 9–23.

Amaratunga, D., Baldry, D., Sarshar, M. & Newton, R. (2002) Quantitative and qualitative research in the built environment: Application of "mixed" research approach. *Work Study*, 51, 17–31.

American Association of Human-Animal Bond Veterinarians (AAHABV) (1998) Statement from the Committee on the Human-Animal. *Journal of the American Veterinary Medical Association*, 212 (11), 1675.

American Veterinary Medical Association [AVMA] (2011) About the AVMA: Who we are. Retrieved from http://www.avma.org/about_avma/whoweare/oath.asp. Accessed 4 August 2012.

Animal Welfare Act (2006) Available at http://www.legislation.gov.uk/ukpga/2006/45/pdfs/ukpga_20060045_en.pdf. Accessed 10 September 2012.

Antelyes, J. (1990) Client hopes, client expectations. *Journal of the American Veterinary Medical Association*, 197, 1596–1597.

APBC (2005) Annual review of cases. http://www.apbc.org.uk/resources/review_2005.pdf. Accessed December 2007.

Animal Welfare in Veterinary Practice, First Edition. James Yeates.
© 2013 Universities Federation for Animal Welfare. Published 2013 by Blackwell Publishing Ltd.

Appleby, D. & Pluijmakers, J. (2003) Separation anxiety in dogs: The function of homeostasis in its development and treatment. *Veterinary Clinics of North America: Small Animal Practice*, **33** (2), 321–344.

Aron, D.N., Palmer, R.H. & Johnson, A.L. (1995) Biologic strategies and a balanced concept for repair of highly comminuted long bone fractures. *Compendium of Continuing Education for the Practicing Veterinarian*, **17**, 35–49.

Asadi-Lari, M., Packham, C. & Gray, D. (2003) Need for redefining needs. *Health and Quality of Life Outcomes*, **1**, 34–39.

Asher, L., Diesel, G., Summers, J.F., McGreevy, P.D. & Collins, L.M. (2009) Inherited defects in pedigree dogs. Part 1: Disorders related to breed standards. *The Veterinary Journal*, **182**, 402–411.

Audi, R. (2006) *Practical Reasoning and Ethical Decision*. Routledge, Oxford, UK.

Austin, E.J., Deary, I.J. & Willock, J. (2001) Personality and intelligence as predictors of economic behaviour in Scottish farmers. *European Journal of Personality*, **15**, S123–S127.

Austin, E.J., Deary, I.J., Edwards-Jones, G. & Arey, D. (2005) Attitudes to farm animal welfare: Factor structure and personality correlates in farmers and agriculture students. *Journal of Individual Differences*, **26**, 107–120.

Azoulay, E., Pochard, F., Chevret, S., *et al.* (2004) Half the family members of intensive care unit patients do not want to share in the decision-making process: A study in 78 French intensive care units. *Critical Care Medicine*, **32** (9), 1832–1838.

Balcombe, J.P. (2006) Laboratory environments and rodents' behavioural needs: A review. *Laboratory Animals*, **40**, 217–235.

Bartussek, H. (2001) An historical account of the development of the animal needs index ANI-35L as part of the attempt to promote and regulate farm animal welfare in Austria: An example of the interaction between animal welfare science and society. *Acta Agriculturae Scandinavica, Section A: Animal Science*, **51** (1S), 34–41.

Bauer, M., Glickman, L., Toombs, J., Golden, S. & Skowronek, C. (1992) Follow-up study of owner attitudes toward home care of paraplegic dogs. *Journal of the American Veterinary Medical Association*, **200**, 1809–1816.

Beach, M.C. & Inui, T.S. (2006) Relationship centered care: A constructive reframing. *Journal of General Internal Medicine*, **21S**, 3–8.

Beerda, B., Schilder, M.B.H., van Hooff, J.A.R.A.M. & de Vries, H.W. (1997) Manifestations of chronic and acute stress in dogs. *Applied Animal Behaviour Science*, **52**, 307–319.

Beerda, B., Schilder, M.B.H., van Hoof, J.A.R.A.M., de Vries, H.W. & Mol, J.A. (1998) Behavioural, saliva cortisol and heart rate responses to different types f stimuli in dogs. *Applied Animal Behaviour Science*, **58**, 365–381.

Beerda, B., Schilder, M.B.H., van Hoof, J.A.R.A.M., de Vries, H.W. & Mol, J.A. (1999) Chronic stress in dogs subjected to social and spatial restriction I. Behavioural responses. *Physiology and Behaviour*, **6** (2), 233–242.

Bengtsson-Tops, A. & Hansson, L. (1999) Clinical and social needs of schizophrenic outpatients living in the community: The relationship between needs and subjective quality of life. *Social Psychiatry and Psychiatric Epidemiology*, **34**, 513–518.

Bennett, R.M., Broom, D.M., Henson, S.J., Blaney, R.J.P. & Harper, G. (2004) Assessment of the impact of government animal welfare policy on farm animal welfare in the UK. *Animal Welfare*, **13**, 1–11.

Bernoulli, D. (1738/1954) Specimen theoriae novae de mensura sortis [Exposition of a new theory on the measurement of risk]. *Econometrica*, **22**, 23–36.

Bessei, W. (2006) Welfare of broilers: A review. *Worlds Poultry Science Journal*, **62**, 455–466.

Blackwell, E., Casey, R. & Bradshaw, J. (2003) The assessment of shelter dogs to predict separation-related behaviour and the validation of advice to reduce its incidence post-homing. RSPCA, Horsham, UK.

Blackwell, E., Casey, R. & Bradshaw, J. (2005) Firework fears and phobias in the domestic dog. RSPCA, Horsham, UK.

Blackwell, M.J. (2001) The 2001 Inverson Bell symposium keynote address: Beyond philo-sophical differences: The future training of veterinarians. *Journal of Veterinary Medical Education*, **28**, 148–152.

Blaxter, M. (1983) The causes of disease: Women talking. *Social Science & Medicine*, **17**, 59–69.

Bock, B.B. & van Huik, M.M. (eds) (2007) Pig farmers and animal welfare: A study of beliefs, attitudes and behaviour of pig farmers across Europe. In: *Attitudes of Consumers, Retailers and Producers to Farm Animal Welfare*, Vol. 2 (eds U. Kjærnes, M. Miele & J. Roex), pp. 73–127. Welfare Quality Reports.

Boissy, A., Arnould, C., Chaillou, E., *et al*. (2007a) Emotions and cognition: A new approach to animal welfare. *Animal Welfare*, **16** (S), 37–43.

Boissy, A., Manteuffel, G., Jensen, M.B., *et al*. (2007b) Assessment of positive emotions in animals to improve their welfare. *Physiology & Behavior*, **92**, 375–397.

Boivin, X., Lensink, J., Tallet, C. & Veissier, I. (2003) Stockmanship and farm animal welfare. *Animal Welfare*, **12**, 479–492.

Bones, V.C. & Yeates, J.Y. (2012) The socio-historical and ethical content of veterinary oaths. *Journal of Animal Ethics*, **2** (1), 20–42.

Borchelt, P.L. & Voith, V.L. (1982) Diagnosis and treatment of separation-related behaviour problems in dogs. *Veterinary Clinics of North America: Small Animal Practice*, **12**, 625–635.

Botreau, R., Veissier, I. & Perny, P. (2009) Overall assessment of animal welfare: Strategy adopted in welfare quality®. *Animal Welfare*, **18**, 363–370.

Bowling, A. (2005) *Measuring Health*, 3rd edn. Open University Press, Maidenhead, UK.

Bracke, M.B.M., Spruijt, B.M. & Metz, J.H.M. (1999) Overall welfare reviewed. Part 3: Welfare assessment based on needs and supported by expert opinion. *Netherland Journal of Agricultural Science*, **47**, 307–322.

Bradley, C. (2001) Importance of differentiating health status from quality of life. *Lancet*, **357**, 7–8.

Bradshaw, J.W.S., McPherson, J.A., Casey, R.A. & Larter, I.S. (2002) Aetiology of separation-related behaviour in domestic dogs. *Veterinary Record*, **151**, 43–46.

Brillard, J.P. (2001) Future strategies for broiler breeders: An international perspective. *Worlds Poultry Science Journal*, **57** (3), 243–250.

Brockman, B.K., Taylor, V.A. & Brockman, C.M. (2008) The price of unconditional love: Consumer decision making for high-dollar veterinary care. *Journal of Business Research*, **61**, 397–405.

Brody, J.E. (2011) Easing the way in therapy with the aid of an animal. *New York Times*, March 14, p. D7.

Brondani, J.T., Luna, S.P.L. & Padovani, C.R. (2011) Refinement and initial validation of a multidimensional composite scale for use in assessing acute postoperative pain in cats. *American Journal of Veterinary Research*, **72**, 174–183.

Broom, D.M. (1999) Animal welfare: The concept of the issues. In: *Attitudes to Animals* (ed. F.L. Dollins), pp. 129–142. Cambridge University Press, Cambridge, UK.

Broom, D.M. (2008) Welfare assessment and relevant ethical decisions: Key concepts. *Annual Reviews in Biomedical Science*, **10**, T79–T90.

Brotherton, I. (1989) Farmer participation in voluntary land diversion schemes: Some observations from theory. *Journal of Rural Studies*, **5**, 299–304.

Brown, C., Thompsong, S., Vroegindeweyg, G. & Pappaioanou, M. (2006) The global veterinarian: The why? The what? The how? *Journal of Veterinary Medical Education*, **33** (3), 411–415.

Brown, J.P. & Silverman, J.P. (1999) The current and future market for veterinarians and veterinary services in the United States. *Journal of the American Veterinary Medical Association*, **215**, 161–183.

Brown, R.M. (1998) Debate regarding tail docking/ear cropping methods. *Journal of the American Veterinary Medical Association*, **213**, 472.

Burn, C.C., Pritchard, J.C. & Whay, H.R. (2009) Observer reliability for working equine welfare assessment: Problems with high prevalences of certain results. *Animal Welfare*, **18**, 177–187.

Bussieres, G., Jacques, C., Lainay, O., *et al.* (2008) Development of a composite orthopaedic pain scale in horses. *Research in Veterinary Science*, **85** (2), 294–306.

Capdeville, J. & Veissier, I. (2001) A method of assessing welfare in loose housed dairy cows at farm level, focusing on animal observations. *Acta Agriculturae Scandinavica, Section A: Animal Science*, S30, 62–68.

Carberry, C.A. & Harvey, H.J. (1997) Owner satisfaction with limb amputation in dogs and cats. *Journal of the American Veterinary Medical Association*, **23**, 227–232.

Catley, A., Blakeway, S. & Leyland, T. (2002) *Community-Based Animal Healthcare*. ITDG Publishing, London, UK.

Chang, P.-C. & Yeh, C.-H. (2005) Agreement between child self-report and parent proxy-report to evaluate quality of life in children with cancer. *Psycho-Oncology*, **14**, 125–134.

Charles, C., Gafni, A. & Whelan, T. (1999) What do we mean by partnership in making decisions about treatment? *British Medical Journal*, **319**, 780–782.

Charon, R. (2006) *Narrative Medicine: Honoring the Stories of Illness*. Oxford University Press, Oxford, UK.

Chester, Z. & Clark, W.T. (1988) Coping with blindness: A survey of 50 blind dogs. *Veterinary Record*, **123**, 668–671.

Colditz, I.G., Walkden-Brown, S.W. & Daly, B.L. (2005) Some physiological responses associated with reduced wool growth during blowfly strike in Merino sheep. *Australian Veterinary Journal*, **11**, 695–699.

Collins, J., Hanlon, A., More, S.J., Wall, P.G. & Duggan, V. (2009) Policy Delphi with vignette methodology as a tool to evaluate the perception of equine welfare. *The Veterinary Journal*, **181**, 63–69.

Companion Animal Welfare Council [CAWC] (2008) *Companion Animal Welfare Surveillance*. CAWC, London, UK.

Companion Animal Welfare Council [CAWC] (2009) *Companion Animal Welfare Assessment*. CAWC, London, UK.

Conselho Federal de Medicina Veterinária [CFMV] (2002) *Resolução n° 722, de 16 de agosto de 2002*. Retrieved from http://www.cfmv.org.br/portal/legislacao/resolucoes/resolucao_722.pdf. Accessed 4 August 2012.

Coppola, C.L., Grandin, T. & Enns, R.M. (2006) Human interaction and cortisol: Can human contact reduce stress for shelter dogs? *Physiology & Behavior*, **87**, 537–541.

Coulter, A. (1999) Paternalism or partnership. *British Medical Journal*, **319**, 719–720.

Craven, M., Simpson, J.W., Ridyard, A.E. & Chandler, M.L. (2004) Canine inflammatory bowel-disease: Retrospective analysis of diagnosis and outcome in 80 cases (1995–2002). *Journal of Small Animal Practice*, **45**, 336–342.

Crespi, L. (1942) Quantitative variation of incentive and performance in the white rat. *American Journal of Psychology*, **55**, 467–517.

Crowell-Davis, S.L., Seibert, L.M., Sung, W., Parthasarathy, V. & Curtis, T.M. (2003) Use of clomopramine, alprazolam and behaviour modification for treatment of storm phobia in dogs. *Journal of the American Veterinary Medical Association*, **222**, 744–748.

Csikszentmihalyi, M. (1999) If we are so rich, why aren't we happy? *American Psychologist*, **54**, 821–827.

Culyer, A. (1998) Need – Is a consensus problem. *Journal of Medical Ethics*, **24**, 77–80.

Curtis, S.E. (1983) Animal well-being and animal care. *Veterinary Clinics of North America: Food Animal Practice*, **3**, 369–382.

Damasio, A. (1995) *Descartes' Error: Emotion, Reason and the Human Brain*. MacMillan, London, UK.

Danbury, T.C., Weeks, C.A., Cambers, J.P., Waterman-Pearson, A.E. & Kestin, S.C. (2000) Self-selection of the analgesic drug carprofen by lame broiler chickens. *Veterinary Record*, **146**, 307–311.

Davison, C., Davey Smith, G. & Frankel, S. (1991) Lay epidemiology and the prevention paradox: The implications of coronary candidacy for health education. *Sociology of Health and Illness*, **13**, 1–19.

De Leeuw, J.A. & Ekkel, E.D. (2004) Effects of feeding level and the presence of a foraging substrate on the behaviour and stress physiological response of individually housed gilts. *Applied Animal Behaviour Science*, **86** (1–2), 15–25.

Decuypere, E., Hocking, P.M., Tona, K., *et al.* (2006) Broiler breeder paradox: A project report. *Worlds Poultry Science Journal*, **62**, 443–453.

DeLisa, J.A. (2002) Quality of life for individuals with SCI: Let's keep up the good work. *Journal of Spinal Cord Medicine*, **25**, 1.

Denton, D.A., McKinley, M.J., Farrell, M. & Egan, G.F. (2009) The role of primordial emotions in the evolutionary origin of consciousness. *Consciousness and Cognition*, **18**, 500–514.

DiMatteo, M.R., Sherbourne, C.D. & Hays, R.D. (1993) Physicians' characteristics influence patient's adherence to medical treatments: Results from the medical outcomes study. *Health Psychology*, **12**, 93–102.

Dollins, F.L. (ed.) (1999) *Attitudes to Animals*. Cambridge University Press, Cambridge, UK.

Dresser, N. (2000) The horse bar mitzvah: A celebratory exploration of the human-animal bond. In: *Companion Animals and Us* (eds A.L. Podbersek, E.S. Paul & J.A. Serpell). Cambridge University Press, Cambridge, UK.

Ducrot, C., Calavas, D., Sabatier, P. & Faye, B. (1998) Qualitative interaction between the observer and the observed in veterinary epidemiology. *Preventive Veterinary Medicine*, **34**, 107–113.

Dunlop, R.H. & Williams, D.J. (1996) *Veterinary Medicine: An Illustrated History*. Mosby-Year Book, Saint Louis, MO.

Edgar, A., Salek, S., Shickle, D. & Cohen, D. (1998) *The Ethical QALY: Ethical Issues in Healthcare Resource Allocations*. Euromed Communications, Haslemere, UK.

Edwards-Jones, G. (2006) Modelling farmer decision-making: Concepts, progress and challenges. *Animal Science*, **82**, 783–790.

Endenberg, N., Hart, H. & de Vries, H.W. (1992) Differences between owners and non-owners of companion animals. *Anthrozoos*, **4** (2), 120–126.

Eurobarometer (2007) *Attitudes of EU Citizens Towards Animal Welfare*. European Commission–DG Agriculture and Rural Development, Brussels.

European Food Safety Authority [EFSA] (2005) Principles of risk assessment of food producing animals: Current and future approaches. Available at http://www.efsa.europa.eu/EFSA/Scientific_Document/comm_summary%20report_scientcoll_4_en.pdf. Accessed 1 February 2010.

European Food Safety Authority [EFSA] (2006) Scientific opinion on the risks of poor welfare in intensive calf farming systems. An update of the Scientific Veterinary Committee Report on the Welfare of Calves. EFSA-Q-2005-014. *The EFSA Journal*, **366**, 1–36. Available at http://www.efsa.europa.eu/en/science/ahaw/ahaw_opinions/1516.html. Accessed 1 February 2010.

Farm Animal Welfare Council [FAWC] (2009) *Farm Animal Welfare in Great Britain: Past, Present and Future*. FAWC, London, UK.

Farmer, T.W. & Mustian, V.M. (1963) Vestibulocerebellar ataxia. A newly defined hereditary syndrome with periodic manifestations. *Archives of Neurology*, **8**, 471–480.

Favrot, C., Linek, M., Mueller, R. & Zini, E. (2010) Development of a questionnaire to assess the impact of atopic dermatitis on health-related quality of life of affected dogs and their owners. *Veterinary Dermatology*, **21**, 64–70.

Fielding, R. (1995) *Clinical Communication Skills*. Hong Kong University Press, Hong Kong.

Fillipich, L.J. (2000) The scientific method. In: *Proceedings of the Avian Health Chapter* (ed. R. Donoley). Australian College of Veterinary Scientists College Science Week, Gold Coast, Australia.

Fine, A.H. (2010) *The Handbook on Animal Assisted Therapy*. Elsevier/Academic Press, Boston, MA.

Firth, A.M. & Haldane, S.L. (1999) Development of a scale to evaluate post-operative pain in dogs. *Journal of the American Veterinary Medical Association*, **214**, 651–659.

Fishbein, M. & Ajzen, I. (1975) *Belief, Attitude, Intention, and Behavior: An Introduction to Theory and Research*. Addison-Wesley, Reading, MA.

Föllmi, J., Steiger, A., Walzer, C., *et al.* (2007) A scoring system to evaluate physical condition and quality of life in geriatric zoo mammals. *Animal Welfare*, **16**, 309–318.

Forbes, N. (2001) Undertaking research in practice 1. Why and what? *In Practice*, **23**, 613–615.

Forbes, N. (2002) Undertaking research in practice 2. How? *In Practice*, **24**, 44–46.

Francione, G. (1994) Animals, property and legal welfarism: "Unnecessary" suffering and the "humane treatment of animals". *Rutgers Law Review*, **46**, 737.

Frankel, R.M. & Stein, T. (1993) The four habits of highly effective clinicians. *The Permanente Journal*, **3** (3), 79–88.

Frankel, R.M., Stein, T. & Krupat, E. (2003) *The Four Habits Approach to Effective Clinical Communication*. Kaiser Permanente, Oakland, CA.

Fraser, D. (1995) Science, values and animal welfare: Exploring the inextricable connection. *Animal Welfare*, **4**, 103–117.

Fraser, D. (2007) *Understanding Animal Welfare: Science in Its Cultural Context*. UFAW/Wiley-Blackwell, London, UK.

Fraser, D. & Duncan, I.J.H. (1998) 'Pleasures', 'pains' and animal welfare: Toward a natural history of affect. *Animal Welfare*, **7**, 383–396.

Freeman, L.M., Rush, J.E. & Farabaugh, A.E. (2005) Development and evaluation of a questionnaire for assessing health related quality of life in dogs with cardiac disease. *Journal of the American Veterinary Medical Association*, **226**, 1864–1868.

Freire, P. (1970/1996) *Pedagogy of the Oppressed*, pp. 136–137. Penguin, London, UK.

Frewer, L.J. & Salter, B. (2002) Public attitudes, scientific advice and the politics of regulatory policy: The case of BSE. *Science and Public Policy*, **29**, 137–145.

Furnham, A. & Heyes, C. (1993) Psychology students' beliefs about animals and animal experimentation. *Personality and Individual Differences*, **15**, 1–10.

German, A.J. (2006) The growing problem of obesity in dogs and cats. *Journal of Nutrition*, **136** (S), 1940–1946.

German, A.J., Holden, S.L., Bissot, T., Hackett, R.M. & Biourge, V. (2007) Dietary energy restriction and successful weight loss in obese client-owned dogs. *Journal of Veterinary Internal Medicine*, **21** (6), 1174–1180.

Gilbert, D. (2006) *Stumbling on Happiness*. Knopf, New York.

Gill, P., Grothey, A. & Loprinzi, C. (2006) Nausea and vomiting in the cancer patient. *Oncology*, 1482–1496.

Glanz, K., Lewis, F.M. & Rimer, B.K. (1997) *Theory at a Glance: A Guide for Health Promotion Practice*. NIH, Bethesda, MD.

Goodwin, R.D. (1975) Trends in the ownership of domestic pets in Great Britain. In: *Pet Animals and Society* (ed. R.S. Anderson), pp. 96–102. Balliere Tindall, London, UK.

Graham, L., Wells, D.L. & Hepper, P.G. (2005) The influence of olfactory stimulation on the behaviour of dogs in a rescue shelter. *Animal Behaviour Science*, **91**, 143–153.

Graham, P.A., Maskell, I.E., Rawlings, J.M., Nash, A.S. & Markwell, P.J. (2002) Influence of a high fibre diet on glycaemic control and quality of life in dogs with diabetes mellitus. *Journal of Small Animal Practice*, **43**, 67–73.

Greenebaum, J. (2004) It's a dog's life: Evaluating from pet to 'fur baby' at yappy hour. *Society and Animals*, **12** (2), 117–135.

Greenhalgh, T. & Hurwitz, B. (eds) (1998) *Narrative Based Medicine*. NMJ Books, London, UK.

Griffiths, T., Giarchi, G., Carr, A., Jones, P. & Horsham, S. (2007) Life-mapping: A 'therapeutic document' approach to needs assessment. *Quality of Life Research*, **16**, 467–481.

Gul, S.T., Ahmad, M., Khan, A. & Hussain, I. (2007) Haemato-biochemical observations in apparently healthy equine species. *Pakistan Veterinary Journal*, **27**, 155–158.

Hall, S.A. (1994) The struggle for the Charter of the Royal College of Veterinary Surgeons. *Veterinary Record*, **134**, 536–540.

Hamlin, M.J., Shearman, J.P. & Hopkins, W.G. (2002) Changes in physiological parameters in overtrained Standardbred racehorses. *Equine Veterinary Journal*, **34**, 383–388.

Hammell, K.W. (2004) Exploring quality of life following high spinal cord injury: A review and critique. *Spinal Cord*, **42**, 491–502.

Harris, J. (1987) QALYfying the value of life. *Journal of Medical Ethics*, **13**, 117–123.

Hart, B.L. (1988) Biological basis of the behaviour of sick animals. *Neuroscience and Biobehavioural Reviews*, **12**, 123–137.

Hartmann, K. & Kuffer, M. (1998) Karnofsky's score modified for cats. *European Journal of Medical Research*, 3, 95–98.

Hastie, R. & Dawes, R.M. (1988) *Rational Choice in an Uncertain World: The Psychology of Judgement and Decision Making*, p. 167. Sage Publications, London, UK.

Hatschbach, P. I. (2006) História da Veterinária. Retrieved from http://www.crmvgo.org.br/index.php?comando=historicoVeterinaria. Accessed 4 August 2012.

Havenstein, G.B., Ferket, P.R. & Qureshi, M.A. (2003) Growth, livability, and feed conversion of 1957 versus 2001 broilers when fed representative 1957 and 2001 broiler diets. *Poultry Science*, 82, 1500–1508.

Hawkins, P. (2002) Recognizing and assessing pain, suffering and distress in laboratory animals: A survey of current practice in the UK with recommendations. *Laboratory Animal*, 36, 378–395.

Heinonen, H., Aro, A.R., Aalto, A.-M. & Uutela, A. (2004) Is the evaluation of the global quality of life determined by emotional status? *Quality of Life Research*, 13, 1347–1356.

Heleski, C.R., Mertig, A.G. & Zanella, A.J. (2005) Results of a national survey of US veterinary college faculty regarding attitudes toward farm animal welfare. *Journal of the American Veterinary Medical Association*, 226 (9), 1538–1546.

Hellyer, P., Rodan, I., Brunt, J., Downing, R., Hagedorn, J.E. & Robertson, S.A. (2007) AAHA/AAFP pain management guidelines for dogs and cats. *Journal of Feline Medicine and Surgery*, 9, 466–480.

Hellyer, P.W. & Gaynor, J.S. (1998) Acute post-surgical pain in dogs and cats. *Compendium of Continuing Education for the Practicing Veterinarian (Small Animals)*, 20, 140–153.

Hemsworth, P.H. (2007) Ethical stockmanship. *Australian Veterinary Journal*, 85 (5), 194–200.

Hemsworth, P.H. & Coleman, G.J. (1998) *Human–Livestock Interactions: The Stockperson and the Productivity and Welfare of Intensively-Farmed Animals*. CAB International, Oxford, UK.

Hennessy, M.B., David, H.N., Williams, M.T., Mellott, C. & Douglas, C.W. (1997) Plasma cortisol levels of dogs at a county animal shelter. *Physiology and Behaviour*, 62, 485–490.

Hennessy, M.B., Williams, M.T., Miller, D.D., Douglas, C.W. & Voith, V.L. (1998) Influence of male and female petters on plasma cortisol and behaviour: Can human interaction reduce the stress of dogs in a public animal shelter? *Applied Animal Behaviour Science*, 61, 63–77.

Hennessy, M.B., Voith, V.L. & Hawke, J.L. (2002) Effects of a program of human animal interaction and alterations in diet composition on activity and hypothalamic-pituitary-adrenal axis in dogs housed in a public animal shelter. *Journal of the American Veterinary Medical Association*, 221, 65–71.

Herzog, H. (2011) The impact of pets on human health and psychological well-being: Fact, fiction, or hypothesis? *Current Directions in Psychological Science*, 20 (4), 236–239.

Herzog, H.A., Vore, T.L. & New, J.C. (1989) Conversations with veterinary students: Attitudes, ethics and animals. *Anthrozoos*, 2, 181–188.

Herzog, H.A., Betchart, N.B. & Pittman, R.D. (1991) Gender, sex role orientation and attitudes towards animals. *Anthrozoos*, 4, 184–191.

Hetts, S.J.D., Clark, J.P. & Calpin, C.E. (1992) Influence of housing conditions on beagle behaviour. *Applied Animal Behaviour Science*, 34, 137–155.

Hewson, C.J. (2006) Veterinarians who swear: Animal welfare and the veterinary oath. *Canadian Veterinary Journal*, 47, 807–811.

Hiby, E.F. (2005) The welfare of kennelled dogs. PhD thesis, University of Bristol.

Hiby, E.F., Rooney, N.J. & Bradshaw, J.W.S. (2004). Dog training methods, their use, effectiveness and interaction with behaviour and welfare. *Animal Welfare*, 13, 63–69.

Higashi, T., Hays, R.D., Brown, J.A., *et al.* (2005) Do proxies reflect patients' health concerns about urinary incontinence and gait problems? *Health and Quality of Life Outcomes*, 3, 75–84.

Hills, A.M. (1993) The motivational bases of attitudes towards animals. *Society and Animals*, 1, 111–128.

Hochbaum, G.M. (1958) *Public Participation in Medical Screening Programmes: A Sociopsychological Study (Public Health Service Publication No. 572).* Government Printing Office, Washington, USA.

Hocking, P.M. (1993) Welfare of broiler breeder and layer females subjected to food and water control during rearing: Quantifying the degree of restriction. *British Poultry Science*, 34, 53–64.

Hocking, P.M. (1996) The role of bodyweight and food intake after photostimulation on ovarian function at first egg in broiler breeder females. *British Poultry Science*, 37, 841–851.

Hocking, P.M. (2004) Measuring and auditing the welfare of broiler breeders. In: *Measuring and Auditing Broiler Welfare* (eds A. Butterworth & C.A. Weeks), pp. 19–36. CABI Publishing, Wallingford, UK.

Hocking, P.M. (2006) High-fibre pelleted rations decrease water intake but do not improve physiological indexes of welfare in food-restricted female broiler breeders. *British Poultry Science*, 47, 19–23.

Hocking, P.M., Waddington, D., Walker, M.A. & Gilbert, A.M. (1989) Control of the development of ovarian follicular hierarchy in broiler breeder pullets by food restriction during rearing. *British Poultry Science*, 30, 161–174.

Hocking, P.M., Maxwell, M.H. & Mitchell, M.A. (1993) Welfare of broiler breeder and layer females subjected to food and water control during rearing. *British Poultry Science*, 34, 443–458.

Hocking, P.M., Maxwell, M.H. & Mitchell, M.A. (1996) Relationships between the degree of food restriction and welfare indices in broiler breeder females. *British Poultry Science*, 37, 263–278.

Hocking, P.M., Maxwell, M.H., Robertson, G.W. & Mitchell, M.A. (2001) Welfare assessment of modified rearing programmes for broiler breeders. *British Poultry Science*, 42, 424–432.

Hocking, P.M., Bernard, R. & Robertson, G.W. (2002) Effects of low dietary protein and different allocations of food during rearing and restricted feeding after peak rate of lay on egg production, fertility and hatchability in female broiler breeders. *British Poultry Science*, 43, 94–103.

Hockly, E., Cordery, P.M., Woodman, B., *et al.* (2002) Environmental enrichment slows disease progression in R6/2 Huntington's disease mice. *Annals of Neurology*, 51, 235–242.

Holloway, L. (2001) Pets and protein: Placing domestic livestock on hobby-farms in England and Wales. *Journal of Rural Studies*, 17, 293–307.

Holmes, M. & Cockroft, P. (2008) *Handbook for Veterinary Clinical Research.* Wiley Blackwell Publishing, Oxford, UK.

Holton, L., Reid, J., Scott, E.M., Pawson, P. & Nolan, A. (2001) Development of a behaviour-based scale to measure acute pain in dogs. *Veterinary Record*, 148, 525–531.

Hosey, G., Melfi, V. & Pankhurst, S. (2009) *Zoo Animals: Behaviour, Management and Welfare.* Oxford University Press, Oxford, UK.

Houpt, K.A. (2011) *Domestic Animal Behaviour for Veterinary Professionals and Animal Scientists.* Wiley-Blackwell, Ames, IA.

Houpt, K.A. & Houpt, T.R. (1989) Social and illumination preferences of mares. *Journal of Animal Science*, **66**, 2159–2164.

Hubrecht, R.C. (1993) A comparison of social and laboratory environmental enrichment methods for laboratory housed dogs. *Applied Animal Behaviour Science*, **37**, 345–361.

Hubrecht, R.C. (1995) Enrichment in puppyhood and its effects on later behaviour of dogs. *Laboratory Animal Science*, **45**, 70–75.

Hudson, J.T., Slater, M.R., Taylor, L., Scott, H.M. & Kerwin, S.C. (2004) Assessing repeatability and validity of a visual analogue scale questionnaire for use in assessing pain and lameness in dogs. *American Journal of Veterinary Research*, **65**, 1634–1643.

Hudson Jones, A. (1998) Narrative in medical ethics. In: *Narrative Based Medicine* (eds T. Greenhalgh & B. Hurwitz), pp. 214–224. NMJ Books, London, UK.

Hurnik, J.F. & Lehman, H. (1988) Ethics and farm animal welfare. *Journal of Agriculture Ethics*, **1**, 305–318.

Illman, J. (2000) *The Expert Patient.* ABPI, London, UK.

International HIV/Aids Alliance (2006) *Tools Together Now.* International HIV/Aids Alliance, Brighton, UK.

Irvine, L. (2003) George's bulldog: What mead's canine companion could have told him about the self. *Sociological Origins*, **3**, 46–49.

Irvine, L. (2007) The question of animal selves: Implications for sociological knowledge and practice. *Qualitative Sociology Review*, **3** (1), 5–22.

Janicke, D.M., Finey, J.W. & Riley, A.W. (2001) Children's health care use: A prospective investigation of factors related to care-seeking. *Medical Care*, **39**, 990–1001.

Jensen, P. & Toates, F.M. (1993) Who needs 'behavioural needs'? Motivational aspects of the needs of animals. *Applied Animal Behaviour Science*, **37**, 161–181.

Jevons, W.S. (1871) *The Theory of Political Economy.* Macmillan, London, UK.

Johnson, R.B. & Onwuegbuzie, A.J. (2004) Mixed methods research: A research paradigm whose time has come. *Educational Researcher*, **33**, 14.

de Jong, I.C., Enting, H., van Voorst, A. & Blokhuis, H.J. (2005) Do low-density diets improve broiler breeder welfare during rearing and laying? *Poultry Science*, **84**, 194–203.

de Jonge, F.H., Tilly, S., Baars, A.M. & Spruijt, B.M. (2008) On the rewarding nature of appetitive feeding behaviour in pigs (*Sus scrofa*): Do domesticated pigs contrafreeload? *Applied Animal Behaviour Science*, **114** (3–4), 359–372.

Jongman, E.C., Morris, J.P., Barnett, J.L. & Hemsworth, P.H. (2000) EEG changes in 4-week-old lambs in response to castration, tail docking, and mulesing. *Australian Veterinary Journal*, **78**, 339–343.

Josephs, R.A., Larrick, R.P., Steele, C.M. & Nisbett, R.E. (1992) Protecting the self from the negative consequences of risky decisions. *Journal of Personality and Social Psychology*, **62**, 26–37.

Jozefiak, T., Larsson, B., Wichstrøm, L., Mattejat, F. & Ravens-Sieberer, U. (2008) Quality of life as reported by school children and their parents: A cross-sectional survey. *Health and Quality of Life Outcomes*, **6**, 34–44.

Julian, R.J. (2005) Production and growth related disorders and other metabolic diseases of poultry: A review. *The Veterinary Journal*, **169**, 350–369.

Kaplan, M.S., Berthelot, J.-M., Feeny, D., McFarland, B.H., Khan, S. & Orpana, H. (2007) The predictive validity of health-related quality of life measures: Mortality in a longitudinal population-based study. *Quality of Life Research*, **16**, 1539–1546.

Kasanen, I.H.E., Sørensen, D.B., Forkman, B. & Sandøe, P. (2010) Ethics of feeding: The omnivore dilemma. *Animal Welfare*, **19**, 37–44.

Kellert, S.R. & Berry, J.K. (1987) Attitudes, knowledge, and behaviours toward wildlife as affected by gender. *Wildlife Society Bulletin*, **15**, 363–371.

Kenney, E. (2004) Pet funerals and animal graves in Japan. *Mortality*, **9**, 1.

Kent, J.E., Molony, V. & Robertson, I.S. (1993) Changes in plasma cortisol concentration in lambs of three ages after three methods of castration and tail docking. *Research in Veterinary Science*, **55**, 246–251.

Keys, A., Brožek, J., Henschel, A., Mickelsen, O. & Taylor, H.L. (1950) *The Biology of Human Starvation*. University of Minnesota Press, Minnesota.

Kidd, A.H., Kidd, R.M. & George, C.C. (1992) Veterinarians and successful pet adoptions. *Psychological Reports*, **66** (3), 551–557.

King, J.N., Simpson, B.S., Overall, K.L., *et al.* (2000) Treatment of separation anxiety in dogs with clomipramine: Results from a prospective, randomised, double-blind, placebo-controlled, parallel-group, multicentre clinical trial. *Applied Animal Behaviour Science*, **67**, 255–275.

King, J.N., Overall, K.L., Appleby, D., *et al.* (2004) Results of a follow-up investigation to a clinical trial testing the efficacy of clomipramine in the treatment of separation anxiety in dogs. *Applied Animal Behaviour Science*, **89**, 233–242.

King, J.S. & Moulton, B. (2006) Rethinking informed consent: The case for shared medical decision-making. *American Journal of Law and Medicine*, **32** (4), 429–501.

Kirkwood, J.K., Sainsbury, A.W. & Bennett, P.M. (1994) The welfare of free-living wild animals: Methods of assessment. *Animal Welfare*, **3**, 257–273.

Kobelt, A.J., Hemsworth, P.H., Barnett, J.L. & Coleman, G.J. (2003) A survey of dog ownership in suburban Australia—Conditions and behaviour problems. *Applied Animal Behaviour Science*, **82**, 137–148.

Koštál, L., Savory, C.J. & Hughes, B.O. (1992) Diurnal and individual variation in behaviour of restricted-fed broiler breeders. *Applied Animal Behaviour Science*, **32**, 361–374.

Kreger, M.D. & Mench, J.A. (1993) Physiological and behavioral effects of handling and restraint in the ball python (*Python regius*) and the blue-tongued skink (*Tiliqua scincoides*). *Applied Animal Behaviour Science*, **38**, 323–336.

Ladd, J.K., Albright, J.L., Beck, A.M. & Ladd, B.T. (1992) Behavioral and physiological studies on the effect of music on animals. *Journal of Animal Science*, **70** (S), 170.

Laing, I.A. (1996) Talking about babies. In: *Talking with Patients* (eds P.R. Myerscough & M. Ford), pp. 142–149. Oxford University Press, Oxford, UK.

Landsberg, G.M., Hunthausen, W. & Ackerman, L. (2003) *Handbook of Behavior Problems of the Dog and Cat*. Saunders, Edinburgh, UK.

Larrick, R.P. & Boles, T.L. (1995) Avoiding regret in decisions with feedback: A negotiation example. *Organizational Behavior and Human Decision Processes*, **63**, 87–97.

Lascelles, B.D.X. & Main, D.C.J. (2002) Surgical trauma and chronically painful conditions—Within our comfort level but beyond theirs? *Journal of the American Veterinary Medical Association*, **221**, 215–222.

Latham, C.E. & Morris, A. (2007) Effects of formal training in communication skills on the ability of veterinary students to communicate with clients. *Veterinary Record*, **160**, 181–186.

LeDoux, J. (1998) *The Emotional Brain.* Weidenfeld & Nicolson, London, UK.

Lee, C. & Fisher, A.D. (2007) Welfare consequences of mulesing of sheep. *Australian Veterinary Journal*, **85**, 89–93.

Lefebvre, D., Diederich, C., Delcourt, M. & Giffroy, J.-M. (2007) The quality of the relation between handler and military dogs influences efficiency and welfare of dogs. *Applied Animal Behaviour Science*, **104**, 49–60.

LePledge, A. & Hunt, S. (1997) The problem of quality-of-life in medicine. *Journal of the American Medical Association*, **278**, 47–50.

Levine, E.D., Ramos, D. & Mills, D.S. (2007) A prospective study of two self help CD based desensitization and counter-conditioning programmes with the use of dog appeasing pheromone for the treatment of firework fears in dogs. *Applied Animal Behaviour Science*, **105**, 311–329.

Lightfoot, J. (1995) Identifying needs and setting priorities: Issues of theory, policy and practice. *Health and Social Care in the Community*, **3**, 105–114.

Lindsay, S.R. (2005) *Handbook of Applied Dog Behaviour and Training*, Vol. 3, Procedures and Protocols. Blackwell Publishing, Ames, IA.

Lloyd, J.W. & King, L.J. (2004) What are the veterinary schools and colleges doing to improve the nontechnical skills, knowledge, aptitudes, and attitudes of veterinary students? *Journal of the American Veterinary Medical Association*, **224**, 1923–1924.

Lloyd, M. & Bor, R. (2004) *Communication Skills for Medicine.* Churchill Livingstone, Edinburgh, UK.

Loveridge, G.G. (1998) Environmental enriched dog housing. *Applied Animal Behaviour Science*, **59**, 101–113.

Lue, T.W., Pantenburg, D.P. & Crawford, P.M. (2008) Impact of the ownerpet and client-veterinarian bond on the care that pets receive. *Journal of the American Veterinary Medical Association*, **232**, 531–540.

Luescher, A.U., McKeow, D.B. & Halip, J. (1991) Stereotypic and obsessive-compulsive disorders in dogs and cats. *Veterinary Clinics of North America: Small Animal Practice*, **21**, 401–413.

Lumsden, J.H., Rowe, R. & Mullen, K. (1980) Hematology and biochemistry reference values for the light horse. *Canadian Journal of Comparative Medicine*, **44**, 32.

Lyubomirsky, S., King, L. & Diener, E. (2005) The benefits of frequent positive affect: Does happiness lead to success? *Psychological Bulletin*, **131**, 803–855.

Main, D.C.J. (2006) Offering the best to patients: Ethical issues associated with the provision of veterinary services. *The Veterinary Record*, **158**, 62–66.

Main, D.C.J., Whay, H.R., Green, L.E. & Webster, J. (2003) Preliminary investigations into the use of expert opinion to compare the overall welfare of dairy cattle farms in different farm assurance schemes. *Animal Welfare*, **12**, 565–569.

Mangione-Smith, R., McGlynn, E.A., Elliott, M.N., Krogstad, P. & Brook, R.H. (1999) The relationship between perceived parental expectations and pediatrician antimicrobial prescribing behavior. *Pediatrics*, **103** (4), 711–718.

Marcus, E. (2005) *Meat Market: Animals, Ethics and Money.* Brio Press, Boston, MA.

Martin, P. & Bateson, P. (1993) *Measuring Behaviour.* Cambridge University Press, Cambridge, UK.

Maslow, A.H. (1943) A theory or human motivation. *Psychological Review*, **50**, 370–396.

Mason, G. (2006) Are wild-born animals 'protected' from stereotypies? In: *Stereotypies in Captive Animals* (eds G. Mason & J. Rushen), 2nd edn. CAB International, Wallingford, UK.

Mason, G. & Mendl, M. (1993) Why is there no simple way of measuring animal welfare? *Animal Welfare*, **2**, 301–319.

Mason, I. (1995) Writing and publishing a paper in a veterinary journal. *Journal of Small Animal Practice*, **36** (5), 214–220.

Maxwell, M.H., Robertson, G.W., Spence, S. & McCorquodale, C.C. (1990) Comparison of haematological values in restricted and ad-libitum fed domestic fowls: White blood cells and thrombocytes. *British Poultry Science*, **31**, 399–405.

Maxwell, M.H., Hocking, P.M. & Robertson, G.W. (1992) Differential leucocyte responses to various degrees of food restriction in broilers, turkeys and ducks. *British Poultry Science*, **33**, 177–187.

Mayo, E. (1933) *The Human Problems of an Industrial Civilization*. MacMillan, New York.

McBride, S.D. & Cuddeford, D. (2001) The putative welfare-reducing effects of preventing equine stereotypic behaviour. *Animal Welfare*, **10**, 173–189.

McCrave, E.A. (1991) Diagnostic criteria for separation anxiety in the dog. *Veterinary Clinics of North America: Small Animal Practice*, **21**, 247–55.

McEarchern, M.G. & Schroeder, M.J.A. (2002) The role of livestock production ethics in consumer values towards meat. *Journal of Agricultural and Environmental Ethics*, **15**, 221–237.

McGreevy, P. (2004) *Equine Behaviour. A Guide for Veterinary Professionals and Equine Scientists*. Saunders, Edinburgh, UK.

McGreevy, P., McLean, A., Buckley, P., McConaghy, F. & McLean, C. (2011) How riding may affect welfare: What the equine veterinary professional needs to know. *Equine Veterinary Education*, **23** (10), 531–539.

McKenzie-Mohr, D. & Smith, W. (1999) *Fostering Sustainable Behaviour*. New Society Publishers, Gabriola Island, BC.

McMillan, F.D. (1998) Rethinking euthanasia: Death as an unintentional outcome. *Journal of the Veterinary Medical Association*, **212**, 1370–1374.

McMillan, F.D. (2002) Development of a mental wellness program for animals. *Journal of the American Veterinary Medical Association*, **220**, 965–972.

McMillan, F.D. (2003) Maximising quality of life in ill animals. *Journal of the American Animal Hospital Association*, **39**, 227–235.

McMillan, F.D. (ed.) (2005) *Mental Health and Well-Being in Animals*. Blackwell Publishing, Ames, IA.

McMillan, F.D. (2007) Predicting quality-of-life outcomes as a guide for decision-making: The challenge of hitting a moving target. *Animal Welfare*, **16**, 135–42.

McMillan, F.D. & Rollin, B.E. (2001) The presence of mind: On reunifying the animal mind and body. *Journal of the American Veterinary Medical Association*, **218** (11), 1723–1727.

Meagher, R.K. (2009) Observer ratings: Validity and value as a tool for animal welfare research. *Applied Animal Behaviour Science*, **119**, 1–14.

Mench, J.A. (1988) The development of aggressive behaviour in male broiler chicks—A comparison with lating-type males and the effect of feed restriction. *Applied Animal Behaviour Science*, **21**, 233–242.

Mench, J.A. (2002) Broiler breeders: Feed restriction and welfare. *World's Poultry Science Journal*, **58**, 23–29.

Miles, S.H. (2004) *The Hippocratic Oath and the Ethics of Medicine*. Oxford University Press, New York.

Millman, S.T. & Duncan, I.J.H. (2000) Effect of male-to-male aggressiveness and feed-restriction during rearing on sexual behaviour and aggressiveness towards females by male domestic fowl. *Applied Animal Behaviour Science*, 70, 63–82.

Mills, D.S., Gandia Estelles, M., Coleshaw, P.H. & Shorthouse, C. (2003) Retrospective analysis of the treatment of fireworks fears in dogs. *Veterinary Record*, 153, 561–562.

Moberg, G.P. (2000) Biological response to stress: Implications for animal welfare. In: *The Biology of Animal Stress* (eds G.P. Moberg & J.A. Mench), pp. 1–21. CABI Publishing, Oxford, UK.

Morgan, K.N. & Tromborg, C.T. (2007) Sources of stress in captivity. *Applied Animal Behaviour Science*, 102, 262–302.

Morton, D. (1992) Docking of dogs: Practical and ethical issues. *Veterinary Record*, 131, 301–306.

Morton, D.B (2007) A hypothetical strategy for the objective evaluation of animal well-being and quality of life using a dog model. *Animal Welfare*, 16, S75–S81.

Mosteller, J. (2008) Animal-companion extremes and underlying consumer themes. *Journal of Business Research*, 61, 512–521.

Mullan, S. & Main, D. (2007) Preliminary evaluation of a quality-of-life screening programme for pet dogs. *Journal of Small Animal Practice*, 48, 314–322.

Mullan, S., Edwards, S.A., Butterworth, A., Ward, M., Wray, H.R. & Main, D.C.J. (2011) Welfare science into practice: A successful case example of working with industry. *Animal Welfare*, 20 (4), 597–611.

Müller-Graf, C., Candiani, D., Barbieri, S., *et al.* (2008) Risk assessment in animal welfare—The EFSA approach. *AATEX*, 14, S789–S794.

Murray, J.K., Browne, W.J., Roberts, M.A., Whitmarsh, A. & Gruffydd-Jones, T.J. (2010) Number and ownership profiles of cats and dogs in the UK. *Veterinary Record*, 166, 163–168.

Myerscough, P.R. & Ford, M. (1996) *Talking with Patients*. Oxford University Press, Oxford, UK.

von Neumann, J. & Morgenstern, O. (1944) *Theory of Games and Economic Behaviour*. Princeton University Press, Princeton, NJ.

New, J.C., Jr., Salman, M.D., King, M., Scarlett, J.M., Kass, P.H. & Hutchinson, J.M. (2000) Characteristics of shelter-relinquished animals and their owners compared with animals and their owners in the U.S. pet-owning households. *Journal of Applied Animal Welfare Science*, 3, 179–201.

Nickerson, R.S. (2008) *Aspects of Rationality*. Psychology Press, New York.

Nijland, M.L., Stam, F. & Seidell, J.C. (2010) Obesity in dogs, but not in cats, is related to obesity in their owners. *Public Health Nutrition*, 23, 1–5.

Nordenfelt, L. (2006) *Animal and Human Health and Welfare: A Comparative Philosophical Analysis*. CABI, Wallingford, UK.

Norton, R.D. & Scheifer, G.W. (1980) Agricultural sector programming models: A review. *European Review of Agricultural Economics*, 7, 229–264.

O'Connor, A.M., Wennberg, J.E., Legare, F., *et al.* (2007) Toward the 'tipping point': Decision aids and informed patient choice. *Health Affairs*, 26 (3), 716–725.

Odendaal, J.S.J. (2000) Animal assisted therapy—Magic or medicine? *Journal of Psychosomatic Research*, 49, 275–280.

O'Farrell, V. (1990) Students' stereotypes of owners and veterinary surgeons. *Veterinary Record*, 127, 625.

Ormerod, E.J. (2008) Bond-centered veterinary practice: Lessons for veterinary faculty and students. *Journal of Veterinary Medical Education*, **35** (4), 545–52.

O'Sullivan, N.P., Dunnington, E.A., Smith, E.J., Gross, W.B. & Siegel, P.B. (1991) Performance of early and late feathering broiler breeder females with different feeding regimes. *British Poultry Science*, **32**, 981–995.

Overall, K. (1997) *Clinical Behavioral Medicine for Small Animals*. Mosby, St Louis, MO.

Pardini, A.U & Katzev, R.D. (1983–1984) The effects of strength of commitment on newspaper recycling. *Journal of Environmental Systems*, **13**, 245–254.

Parker, D., Stradling, S.G. & Manstead, A.S.R. (1996) Modifying beliefs and attitudes toward exceeding the speed limit: An intervention study based on the theory of planned behavior. *Journal of Applied Social Psychology*, **26**, 1–19.

Parker, R.A. & Yeates, J. (2012) Assessment of quality of life in equine patients. *Equine Veterinary Journal*, **44** (2), 244–249.

Passineau, M.J., Green, E.J. & Dietrich, W.D. (2001) Therapeutic effects of environmental enrichment on cognitive function and tissue integrity following severe traumatic brain injury in rats. *Experimental Neurology*, **168**, 373–384.

Patronek, G.J., Glickman, L.T., Beck, A.M., McCabe, G.P. & Ecker, C. (1996) Risk factors for relinquishment of dogs to an animal shelter. *Journal of the American Veterinary Medical Association*, **209** (3), 572–581.

Paul, E.S. & Podberscek, A.L. (2000) Veterinary education and students' attitudes towards animal welfare. *Veterinary Record*, **146**, 269–272.

PDSA (2010) Long live pets. http://www.pdsa.org.uk/resources/yrp_v11.swf?d= 1291082808.

PDSA (2011) PDSA animal wellbeing report. http://www.pdsa.org.uk/pet-health-advice/ pdsa-animal-wellbeing-report?animal=dog.

Peers, A., Mellor, D.J., Wintour, E.M. & Dodic, M. (2002) Blood pressure, heart rate, hormonal and other acute responses to rubber-ring castration and tail docking of lambs. *New Zealand Veterinary Journal*, **50**, 56–62.

Penticuff, J. & Arheart, K. (2005) Effectiveness of an intervention to improve parent-professional collaboration in neonatal intensive care. *Journal of Perinatal and Neonatal Nursing*, **19** (2), 187–202.

Petrie, A. & Watson, P. (1999) *Statistics for Veterinary and Animal Science*. Blackwell Science, Oxford, UK.

Phillips, C.J.C. (2009) A review of mulesing and other methods to control flystrike (cutaneous myiasis) in sheep. *Animal Welfare*, **18**, 113–121.

Podberscek, A.L., Hsu, Y. & Serpell, J.A. (1999) Evaluation of clomipramine as an adjunct to behavioural therapy in the treatment of separation-related problems in dogs. *Veterinary Record*, **145**, 365–369.

Porter, D.G. (1992) Ethical scores for animal experiments. *Nature*, **356**, 101–102.

Potter, C. & Gasson, R. (1988) Farmer participation in voluntary land diversion schemes: Some predictions from a survey. *Journal of Rural Studies*, **4**, 365–375.

Potthoff, A. & Carithers, R.W. (1989) Pain and analgesia in dogs and cats. *Compendium of Continuing Veterinary Education*, **11**, 887–896.

Pressman, S. & Cohen, S. (2005) Does positive affect influence health? *Psychological Bulletin*, **131**, 925–971.

Prieto, P. & Sacristán, J.A. (2003) Problems and solutions in calculating quality-adjusted life years (QALYs). *Health and Quality of Life Outcomes*, **1**, 80.

Pritchard, J.C., Lindberg, A.C., Main, D.C.J. & Whay, H.R. (2005) Assessment of the welfare of working horses, mules and donkeys, using health and behaviour parameters. *Preventive Veterinary Medicine*, **69**, 265–283.

Radford, A.D., Stockley, P., Taylor, I.R., *et al.* (2003) Use of simulated clients in training veterinary undergraduates in communication skills. *Veterinary Record*, **152**, 422–427.

Radford, M. (2001) *Animal Welfare Law in Britain: Regulation and Responsibility*. Oxford University Press, Oxford.

Reid, J., Nolan, A.M., Hughes, J.M.L., Lascelles, D., Pawson, P. & Scott, E.M. (2007) Development of the short-form Glasgow Composite Measure Pain Scale (CMPS-SF) and derivation of an analgesic intervention score. *Animal Welfare*, **16** (S), 97–104.

Renema, R.A., Rustad, M.E. & Robinson, F.E. (2007) Implications of changes to commercial broiler and broiler breeder body weight targets over the past 30 years. *World's Poultry Science Journal*, **63**, 457–472.

Ritov, I. (1996) Probability of regret: Anticipation of uncertainty resolution in choice. *Organizational Behavior and Human Decision Processes*, **66**, 228–236.

Robert, S., Rushen, J. & Farmer, C. (1997) Both energy content and bulk of food affect stereotypic behaviour, heart rate and feeding motivation of female pigs. *Applied Animal Behaviour Science*, **54**, 161–171.

Robinson, D.A., Romans, C.W., Gordon-Evans, W.J., Evans, R.B. & Conzemius, M.G. (2007) Evaluation of short-term limb function following unilateral carbon dioxide laser or scalpel onychectomy in cats. *Journal of the American Veterinary Medical Association*, **230**, 353–358.

Robson, P.J., Alston, T.D. & Myburgh, K.H. (2003) Prolonged suppression of the innate immune system in the horse following an 80 km endurance race. *Equine Veterinary Journal*, **35**, 133–137.

Rollin, B.E. (2006a) *An Introduction to Veterinary Medical Ethics*. Blackwell, Ames, IA.

Rollin, B.E. (2006b) Euthanasia and quality of life. *Journal of the American Veterinary Medical Association*, **228** (7), 1014–1016.

Rooney, N.J., Gaines, S.A. & Bradshaw, J.W.S. (2007) Behavioural and glucocorticoid responses of dogs (*Canis familiaris*) to kennelling: Investigating mitigating stress by prior habituation. *Physiology & Behaviour*, **92**, 847–854.

Rooney, N., Gaines, S. & Hiby, E (2009) A practitioner's guide to working dog welfare. *Journal of Veterinary Behavior*, **4**, 127–134.

Rosenstock, I. (1974) Historical origins of the health belief model. *Health Education Monographs*, **2** (4), 328–335.

Rosenstock, I.M., Strecher, V.J. & Becker, M.H. (1988) Social learning theory and the health belief model. *Health Education Quarterly*, **15** (2), 175–183.

Roter, D.L. (2000) The enduring and evolving nature of the patient-physician relationship. *Patient Education Counselling*, **39**, 5–15.

Royal Society for the Prevention of Cruelty to Animals [RSPCA] (2008) *The Welfare State: Measuring Animal Welfare in the UK*. RSPCA, Horsham, UK.

Rumsfeld, J.S., MaWhinney, S., McCarthy, M., *et al.* (1999) Health-related quality of life as a predictor of mortality following coronary artery bypass graft surgery. *Journal of the American Medical Association*, **281**, 1298–1303.

Rutherford, K.M.C. (2002) Assessing pain in animals. *Animal Welfare*, **11**, 31–53.

Salman, M.D., New, J.G., Scarlett, J.M. & Kris, P.H. (1998) Human and animal factors related to the relinquishment of dogs and cats in 12 selected animal shelters in the United States. *Journal of Applied Animal Welfare*, **1**, 207–226.

Salman, M.D., Hutchison, J. & Ruch-Gallie, R. (2000) Behavioral reasons for relinquishment of dogs and cats to 12 shelters. *Journal of Applied Animal Welfare Science*, **3**, 93–106.

Sanders, C., Eggerm, M., Donovan, J., Tallon, D. & Frankel, S. (1998) Reporting on quality of life in randomised controlled trials: Bibliographic study. *British Medical Journal*, **317**, 1191–1194.

Sandford, J., Ewbank, R., Molony, V., Tavernor, W.D. & Uvarov, O. (1986) Guidelines for the recognition and assessment of pain in animals. *The Veterinary Record*, **118**, 334–338.

Savage, L.J. (1954) *The Foundations of Statistics.* Wiley, New York.

Savory, C.J., Seawright, E. & Watson, A. (1992) Stereotyped behaviour in broiler breeders in relation to husbandry and opioid receptor blockade. *Applied Animal Behaviour Science*, **32**, 349–360.

Savory, C.J. & Maros, K. (1993) Influence of degree of food restriction, age and time on behaviour of broiler breeder chicks. *Behavioural Processes*, **29**, 179–190.

Savory, C.J., Maros, K. & Rutter, S.M. (1993a) Assessment of hunger in growing broiler breeders in relation to a commercial restricted feeding programme. *Animal Welfare*, **2**, 131–152.

Savory, C.J., Carlisle, A., Maxell, M.H., Mitchell, M.A. & Robertson, G.W. (1993b) Stress, arousal and opioid peptide-like immunoreactivity in restricted and ad lib fed broiler breeder fowls. *Comparative Biochemistry and Physiology*, **106A**, 587–594.

Savory, C.J., Hocking, P.M., Mann, J.S. & Maxwell, M.H. (1996) Is broiler breeder welfare improved by using qualitative rather than quantitative food restriction to limit growth rate? *Animal Welfare*, **5**, 105–127.

Savory, C.J. & Mann, J.S. (1999) Stereotyped pecking after feeding by restricted-fed fowls is influenced by meal size. *Applied Animal Behaviour Science*, **62**, 209–217.

Savory, C.J. & Lariviere, J.-M. (2000) Effects of qualitative and quantitative food restriction treatments on feeding motivational state and general activity level of growing broiler breeders. *Applied Animal Behaviour Science*, **69**, 135–147.

SCAHAW (2000) The welfare of chickens kept for meat production (broilers). *Scientific Committee on Animal Health And Animal Welfare.* European Commission, Health and Consumer Protection Directorate-General.

Scarlett, J.M., Salman, M.D., New, J.G. & Kass, P.H. (2002) The role of veterinary practitioners in reducing dog and cat relinquishments and euthanasias. *Journal of the American Veterinary Medical Association*, **220** (3), 306–311.

Seligman, C. & Darley, J.M. (1977) Feedback as a means of decreasing residential energy consumption. *Journal of Applied Psychology*, **62**, 363–368.

Sepucha, K.R., Fowler, F.J., Jr. & Mulley, A.G., Jr. (2004) Policy support for patient-centered care: The need for measurable improvements in decision quality. *Health Affairs*, **23**, 54–62.

Serpell, J.A. (1996) Evidence for an association between pet behaviour and owner attachment levels. *Applied Animal Behaviour Science*, **47**, 49–60.

Sharp, J.L., Zammit, T.G., Azar, T.A. & Lawson, D.M. (2002) Stress-like responses to common procedures in male rats housed alone or with other rats. *Contemporary Topics in Laboratory Animal Science*, **41**, 8–14.

Shaw, J., Adams, C., Bonnett, B., *et al.* (2004) Use of the Roter interaction analysis system to analyze veterinarian-client-patient communication in companion animal practice. *Journal of the American Veterinary Medical Association*, **225**, 222–229.

Shaw, J.R., Bonnett, B.N., Adams, C.L, *et al.* (2006) Veterinarian-client-patient communication patterns used during clinical appointments in companion animal practice. *Journal of the American Veterinary Medical Association*, **228**, 714–721.

Shaw, J.R., Adams, C.L., Bonnett, B.N., Larson, S. & Roter, D.L. (2008) Veterinarian-client-patient communication during wellness appointments versus appointments related to a health problem in companion animal practice. *Journal of the American Veterinary Medical Association*, **233** (10), 1576–1586.

Sheppard, G. & Mills, D.S. (2003) Evaluation of dog-appeasing pheromone as a potential treatment for dogs fearful of fireworks. *Veterinary Record*, **152**, 432–436.

Sherman, B.L. & Mills, D.S. (2008) Canine anxieties and phobias: An update on separation anxiety and noise aversions. *Veterinary Clinics of North America: Small Animal Practice*, **38**, 1081–1106.

Shutt, D.A., Fell, L.R., Connell, R., Bell, A.K., Wallace, C.A. & Smith, A.I. (1987) Stress-induced changes in plasma concentrations of immunoreactive β-endorphin and cortisol in response to routine surgical procedures in lambs. *Australian Journal of Biological Science*, **40**, 97–103.

Silverman, J., Kurtz, S. & Draper, J. (2005) *Skills for Communicating with Patients*. Radcliffe Medical Press, Oxford, UK.

Simpson, B.S. (1997) Canine communication. *Veterinary Clinics of North America: Small Animal Practice*, **27**, 445–464.

Siracusa, C., Manteca, X., Cerón, J., *et al.* (2008) Perioperative stress response in dogs undergoing elective surgery: Variations in behavioural, neuroendocrine, immune and acute phase responses. *Animal Welfare*, **17**, 259–273.

Slater, M.R., Robinson, L.E., Zoran, D.L., Wallace, K.A. & Scarlett, J.M. (1995) Diet and exercise patterns in pet dogs. *Journal of the American Veterinary Medical Association*, **207**, 186–190.

Slater, M.R., Di Nardo, A., Pediconi, O., *et al.* (2008) Cat and dog ownership and management patterns in central Italy. *Preventive Veterinary Medicine*, **85**, 267–294.

Spinelli, J.S. & Markowitz, H. (1987) Clinical recognition and anticipation of situations likely to induce suffering in animals. *Journal of the American Veterinary Medical Association*, **191**, 1216–1218.

SPVS/PDF Clinical Audit Group (2007) *Guide to Clinical Audit: Improving Clinical Effectiveness in Veterinary Practice through the Introduction of Clinical Audit*. SPVS, Warwick, UK.

Stacey, M. (1994) The power of lay knowledge: A personal view. In: *Researching the People's Health* (eds J. Popay & G. Williams). Routledge, London, UK.

Stein, T., Frankel, R.M. & Krupat, E. (2005) Enhancing clinician communication skills in a large healthcare organization: A longitudinal case study. *Patient Education and Counseling*, **58**, 4–12.

Stewart, M.A. (1995) Effective physician-patient communication and health outcomes: A review. *Canadian Medical Association Journal*, **152**, 1423–1433.

Stimson, G.V. (1974) Obeying the doctor's orders: A view from the other side. *Social Science & Medicine*, **8**, 97–104.

Suh, E.M., Diener, E. & Fujita, F. (1996) Events and subjective well-being: Only recent events matter. *Journal of Personality and Social Psychology*, 70, 1091–1102.

Summers, J.F., Diesel, G., Asher, L., McGreevy, P.D. & Collins, L.M. (2010) Inherited defects in pedigree dogs. Part 2: Disorders that are not related to breed standards. *The Veterinary Journal*, 183, 39–45.

Swabe, J. (1999). *Animals, Disease and Human Society: Human-Animal Relations and the Rise of Veterinary Medicine*. Routledge Studies in Science, Technology and Society, London, UK.

Tadich, N., Mendez, G., Wittwer, F. & Meyer, K. (1997) Valores bioquímicos sanguíneos de equinos que tiran carretones en la ciudad de Valdivia (Chile) (Blood biochemical values of loadcart draught horses in the city of Valdivia (Chile)). *Archivos de Medicina Veterinaria*, 29, 45–53.

Takeuchi, Y., Ogata, N., Houpt, K.A. & Scarlett, J.M. (2001) Differences in background and outcome of three behavior problems of dogs. *Applied Animal Behaviour Science*, 70, 297–308.

Tannenbaum, J. (1993) Veterinary medical ethics: A focus of conflicting interests. *Journal of Social Issues*, 49 (1), 143–156.

Tannenbaum, J. (1995) Animals and the law: Cruelty, property, rights... or how the law makes up in common sense what it may lack in metaphysics. *Social Research*, 62 (3), 539–607.

Tate, P. (2003) *The Doctor's Communication Handbook*. Radcliffe Medical Press Ltd, Oxford, UK.

Taylor, A.A. & Weary, D.M. (2000) Vocal response of piglets to castration: Identifying procedural sources of pain. *Applied Animal Behaviour Science*, 70, 17–26.

Taylor, D., Bury, M., Campling, N., *et al.* (2007) A review of the use of the health belief model (HBM), the theory of reasoned action (TRA), the theory of planned behaviour (TPB) and the trans-theoretical model (TTM) to study and predict health-related behaviour change. NHS National Institute for Health and Clinical Excellence (NICE). Available at http://www2.warwick.ac.uk/fac/med/study/ugr/mbchb/phase1_08/semester2/healthpsychology/nice-doh_draft_review_of_health_behaviour_theories.pdf. Accessed 5 July 2011.

Taylor, N. (2007) Never an it: Intersubjectivity and the creation of animal personhood in animal shelters. *Qualitative Sociology Review*, 3 (1), 59–73.

Taylor, P.M. & Robertson, S.A. (2004) Pain management in cats: Past, present and future. Part 1. The cat is unique. *Journal of Feline Medicine and Surgery*, 6, 313–320.

Tetlock, P.E. & Boettger, R. (1994) Accountability amplifies the status quo effect when change creates victims. *Journal of Behavioral Decision Making*, 7, 1–23.

Thornton, P.D. & Waterman-Pearson, A.E. (2002) Behavioural responses to castration in lambs. *Animal Welfare*, 11, 203–212.

Thrusfield, M. (1995) *Veterinary Epidemiology*. Blackwell Science, Oxford, UK.

Timmins, R.P., Cliff, K.D., Day, C.T., *et al.* (2007) Enhancing quality of life for dogs and cats in confined situations. *Animal Welfare*, 16 (S), 83–87.

Tischler, J. (1977) Rights for non-human animals. A guardianship model for dogs and cats. *San Diego Law Review*, 14, 484–506.

Tourangeau, R. & Yan, T. (2007) Sensitive questions in surveys. *Psychological Bulletin*, 133, 859–883.

Tovey, P. (1998) Narrative and knowledge development in medical ethics. *Journal of Medical Ethics*, 24, 176–181.

Tuber, D.S., Hennessy, M.B., Sanders, S. & Miller, J.A. (1996) Behavioral and glucocorticoid responses of adult domestic dogs (*Canis familiaris*) to companionship and social separation. *Journal of Comparative Psychology*, **110** (1), 103–108.

Tuber, D.S., Miller, D.D., Caris, R.H., Halter, R., Linden, F. & Hennessy, M.B. (1999) Dogs in animal shelters: Problems, suggestions and needed expertise. *Psychological Science*, **10**, 379–386.

Tzannes, S., Hammond, M.F., Murphy, S., Sparkes, A. & Blackwood, L. (2008) Owners' perception of their cats' quality of life during COP chemotherapy for lymphoma. *Journal of Feline Medicine and Surgery*, **10**, 73–81.

Ubel, P.A., Loewenstein, G., Schwarz, N. & Smith, N. (2005) Misimagining the unimaginable: The disability paradox and health care decision-making. *Health Psychology*, **24**, S57–S62.

Vaarst, M., Nissen, T.B., Østergaard, S., Klaas, I.C., Bennedsgaard, T.W. & Christensen, J. (2007) Danish stable schools for experiential common learning in groups of organic dairy farmers. *Journal of Dairy Science*, **90**, 2543–2554.

Vanslembrouck, I., Van Huylenbroeck, G. & Verbeke, W. (2002) Determinants of the willingness of Belgian farmers to participate in agri-environmental measures. *Journal of Agricultural Economics*, **53**, 489–511.

Varni, J.W., Limbers, C.A. & Burwinkle, T.M. (2007) Parent proxy-report of their children's health-related quality of life: An analysis of 13,878 parents' reliability and validity across age subgroups using the PedsQL™ 4.0 Generic Core Scales. *Health & Quality of Life Outcomes*, **5**, 2–11.

Velde, H.T., Aarts, N. & Van Woerkum, C. (2002) Dealing with ambivalence: Farmers' and consumers' perceptions of animal welfare in livestock breeding. *Journal of Agricultural and Environmental Ethics*, **15**, 203–219.

Verbeke, W.A.J. & Viaene, J. (2000) Ethical challenges for livestock production: Meeting consumer concerns about meat safety and animal welfare. *Journal of Agricultural and Environmental Ethics*, **12**, 141–151.

Visser, E.K., Ellis, A.D. & Van Reenen, C.G. (2008) The effect of two different housing conditions on the welfare of young horses stabled for the first time. *Applied Animal Behaviour Science*, **114**, 521–533.

Waldau, P. (2011) *Animal Rights: What Everyone Needs to Know*. Oxford University Press, Oxford, UK.

Wallace, M.T. & Moss, J.E. (2002) Farmer decision-making with conflicting goals: A recursive strategic programming analysis. *Journal of Agricultural Economics*, **53**, 82–100.

Wathes, C. (2010) Lives worth living? *Veterinary Record*, **166**, 468–469.

Wayner, C.J. & Heinke, M.L. (2006) Compliance: Crafting quality care. *Veterinary Clinics of North America: Small Animal Practice*, **36** (2), 419–436.

Webster, J. (1994) *Animal Welfare: A Cool Eye Towards Eden*. Blackwell, Oxford, UK.

Webster, J. (2005) *Animal Welfare: Limping Towards Eden*. Blackwell, Oxford, UK.

Weiss, M. & Britten, N. (2003). What is concordance? *Pharmaceutical Journal*, **271**, 493.

Wells, D.L. (2004) A review of environmental enrichment for kennelled dogs, *Canis familiaris*. *Applied Animal Behaviour Science*, **85**, 307–317.

Wells, D.L. & Hepper, P.G. (1992) The behaviour of dogs in a rescue shelter. *Animal Welfare*, **1**, 171–186.

Wells, D.L. & Hepper, P.G. (1998) A note on the influence of visual conspecific contact on the behaviour of sheltered dogs. *Applied Animal Behaviour Science*, **60**, 83–88.

Wells, D.L. & Hepper, P.G. (1999) Male and female dogs respond differently to men and women. *Applied Animal Behaviour Science*, **68**, 151–162.

Wells, D.L. & Hepper, P.G. (2000) The influence of environmental change on the behaviour of sheltered dogs. *Applied Animal Behaviour Science*, **68**, 151–162.

Wells, D.L., Graham, L. & Hepper, P.G. (2002) The influence of auditory stimulation on the behaviour of dogs housed in a rescue shelter. *Animal Welfare*, **11**, 385–393.

Wemelsfelder, F. (1997) The scientific validity of subjective concepts in models of animal welfare. *Applied Animal Behaviour Science*, **53**, 75–88.

Wemelsfelder, F. (2007) How animals communicate quality of life: The qualitative assessment of behaviour. *Animal Welfare*, **16** (S), 25–31.

Wemelsfelder, F., Hunter, T.E.A., Mendl, M.T. & Lawrence, A.B. (2001) Assessing the 'whole animal': A free choice profiling approach. *Animal Behaviour*, **62** (2), 209–220.

Wennberg, J.E. (2002) Unwarranted variations in healthcare delivery: Implications for academic medical centres. *British Medical Journal*, **325** (7370), 961–964.

Wensley, S.P. (2008) Animal welfare and the human-animal bond, considerations for veterinary faculty, students, and practitioners. *Journal of Veterinary Medical Education*, **35** (4), 532–539.

Westgarth, C., Pinchbeck, G.L., Bradshaw, J.W.S., Dawson, S., Gaskell, R.M. & Christley, R.M. (2007) Factors associated with dog ownership and contact with dogs in a UK community. *BMC Veterinary Research*, **3**, 5.

Whay, H.R., Main, D.C.J., Green, L.E. & Webster, J. (2003) Animal-based measures for the assessment of welfare state of dairy cattle, pigs and laying hens: Consensus of expert opinion. *Animal Welfare*, **12** (4), 611–617.

Whitehead, C.C., Herron, K.M. & Waddington, D. (1987) Reproductive performance of dwarf broiler breeders given different food allowances during the rearing and breeding periods on two lighting patterns. *British Poultry Science*, **28**, 415–427.

Whiteneck, G.G., Charlifue, S.W., Frankel, H.L., *et al.* (1992) Mortality, morbidity, and psychosocial outcomes of persons spinal cord injured more than 20 years ago. *Paraplegia*, **30**, 617–630.

Williams, G. & Popay, J. (2006) Lay knowledge and the privilege of experience. In: *Challenging Medicine* (eds J. Gabe, D. Kelleher & G. Williams), pp. 118–139. Routledge, London, UK.

Willis, N.G., Monroe, F.A., Potworowski, J.A., *et al.* (2007) Envisioning the future of veterinary medical education: The Association of American Veterinary Medical Colleges Foresight Project, final report. *Journal of Veterinary Medical Education*, **34** (1), 1–41.

Willock, J., Deary, I.J., McGregor, M.J., *et al.* (1999a) Farmers' attitudes, objectives, behaviours and personality traits. The Edinburgh study of decision making on farms. *Journal of Vocational Behaviour*, **54**, 5–36.

Willock, J., Deary, I., Edwards-Jones, G., *et al.* (1999b) The role of attitudes and objectives in farmer decision-making: Business and environmentally oriented behaviour in Scotland. *Journal of Agricultural Economics*, **50**, 286–303.

Winberg, B., Jensen, A.J., Johanssen, P.I., *et al.* (2010) Developing a scoring system for disseminated intravascular coagulation in dogs. *Veterinary Journal*, **185**, 292–298.

Wiseman-Orr, M.L., Nolan, A.M., Reid, J. & Scott, E.M. (2004) Development of a questionnaire to measure the effects of chronic pain on health-related quality of life in dogs. *American Journal of Veterinary Research*, **65**, 1077–1084.

Wiseman-Orr, M.L, Scott, E.M., Reid, J. & Nolan, A.M. (2006) Validation of a structured questionnaire as an instrument to measure chronic pain in dogs on the basis of effects on health-related quality of life. *American Journal of Veterinary Research*, 67, 1826–1836.

Wiseman-Orr, M.L., Scott, E.M. & Nolan, A.M. (2011a) Development and testing of a novel instrument to measure health-related quality-of-life (HRQL) of farmed pigs and promote welfare enhancement (Part 1). *Animal Welfare*, 20 (4), 535–548.

Wiseman-Orr, M.L., Scott, E.M. & Nolan, A.M. (2011b) Development and testing of a novel instrument to measure health-related quality-of-life (HRQL) of farmed pigs and promote welfare enhancement (Part 2). *Animal Welfare*, 20 (4), 549–558.

Withrow, S.J. & Hirsch, V.M. (1979) Owner response to amputation of a pet's leg. *Veterinary Medicine—Small Animal Clinician*, 74, 332–4.

Wojciechowska, J.I. & Hewson, C.J. (2005) Quality-of-life-assessment in pet dogs. *Journal of the American Veterinary Medical Association*, 226, 722–728.

Wojciechowska, J.I., Hewson, C.J., Stryhn, H., Guy, N.C., Patronek, G.J. & Timmons, V. (2005). Development of a discriminative questionnaire to assess nonphysical aspects of quality of life of dogs. *American Journal of Veterinary Research*, 66, 1453–1460.

Wolfensohn, S. & Honess, P. (2007) Laboratory animal, pet animal, farm animal, wild animal: Which gets the best deal? *Animal Welfare*, 16 (S), 117–123.

Wyse, C.A., McNie, K.A., Tannahil, V.J., Murray, J.K. & Love, S. (2008) Prevalence of obesity in riding horses in Scotland. *Veterinary Record*, 162, 590–591.

Yeates, J. (2009a) Response and responsibility: An analysis of veterinary ethical conflicts. *The Veterinary Journal*, 182 (1), 3–6.

Yeates, J. (2009b) Death is a welfare issue. *Journal of Agricultural and Environmental Ethics*, 23 (3), 229–240.

Yeates, J. (2010a) The value of pleasure and pain in welfare ethics. *Animal Welfare*, 19 (S), 29–38.

Yeates, J. (2010b) When to euthanase. *Veterinary Record*, 166, 370–371.

Yeates, J. (2010c) Ethical aspects of euthanasia of owned animals. *In Practice*, 32, 70–73.

Yeates, J. (2011a) The application of veterinary stem cell technologies to dogs and horses. In: *Bioethics and the Global Politics of Stem Cell Science: Medical Applications in a Pluralistic World* (eds A.V. Campbell & B.C. Capps). Imperial College Press/World Scientific Publishing Co, London, UK.

Yeates, J. (2011b) Is 'a life worth living' a concept worth having? *Animal Welfare*, 20, 397–406.

Yeates, J. (2012a) Dog welfare from a veterinary perspective. *The Veterinary Journal*, 192 (3), 272–278.

Yeates, J. (2012b) Quality time: Ethical approaches to the 'life worth living' concept in farm animal welfare. *Journal of Agricultural and Environmental Ethics*, 25 (4), 607–624.

Yeates, J. (2012c) Whistleblowing in the veterinary profession. *The Veterinary Journal*, 191, 147–150.

Yeates, J. (2012d) Economics and animal welfare: The case of dog breeding. *UFAW*, 21 (S1), 155–160.

Yeates, J. & Main, D.C.J. (2008) Positive welfare: A review. *The Veterinary Journal*, 175, 293–300.

Yeates, J. & Main, D.C.J. (2009) Assessment of companion animal QOL in research and practice. *Journal of Small Animal Practice*, 50 (6), 274–281.

Yeates, J. & Main, D.C.J. (2010) The ethics of influencing clients: Problems and solutions. *Journal of the American Veterinary Medical Association*, **237** (3), 263–267.

Yeates, J. & Main, D.C.J. (2011a) Veterinary surgeons' opinions on dog welfare issues. *Journal of Small Animal Practice*, **52** (9), 464–468.

Yeates, J. & Main, D.C.J. (2011b) Veterinary opinions on refusing euthanasia: Justifications and philosophical frameworks. *Veterinary Record*, **168**, 263–265.

Yeates, J., Mullen, S., Stone, M. & Main, D.C.J. (2011) Promoting discussions and decisions about dogs' quality of life. *Journal of Small Animal Practice*, **52** (9), 459–463.

Young, R.J. (1999) The behavioural requirements of farm animals for psychological well-being and survival. In: *Attitudes to Animals* (ed. F.L. Dollins), pp. 77–100. Cambridge University Press, Cambridge, UK.

Zanella, R., Heleski, C. & Zanella, A.J. (2003) Assessment of the Michigan State University equine welfare intervention strategy (MSU-EQWIS-ACTION) using Brazilian draught horses as a case study. In: *Proceedings of the 37th International Congress of the International Society for Applied Ethology*, Abano Terme, Italy, 24–28 June, p. 192.

Index

Animal Welfare in Veterinary Practice, First Edition. James Yeates.
© 2013 Universities Federation for Animal Welfare. Published 2013 by Blackwell Publishing Ltd.